10.99

pilates for pregnancy

pilates for pregnancy

michael king
and yolande green

MITCHELL BEAZLEY

pilates for pregnancy
Michael King and Yolande Green

Published in 2002 by Mitchell Beazley, an imprint of
Octopus Publishing Group Limited,
2–4 Heron Quays, London E14 4JP

ISBN 1 84000 540 8
A CIP catalogue record for this book is available from the British Library

Publisher's note: Before following any advice or exercises contained in this book, it is
recommended that you consult your doctor if you suffer from any health problems or special
conditions. The publishers cannot accept responsibility for any injuries or damage incurred as
a result of following the advice given in this book.

Executive Editors: Vivien Antwi, Lindsay Porter
Executive Art Editor: Christine Keilty
Project Editor: Naomi Waters
Editor: Mary Loebig Giles
Design: cobalt*id*
Proofreader: Siobhan O'Connor
Production: Angela Couchman
Photography: Ruth Jenkinson
Models: Emma Buckle, Melanie Campbell, Claire Lyons, Rebecca Rochford Davies

Typeset in Kepler and Franklin Gothic
Printed and bound by Toppan Printing Company, China

If you would like further information about Pilates courses, training, workshops or classes,
please contact The Pilates Institute on 020 7253 3177 or visit www.pilates-institute.co.uk.

contents

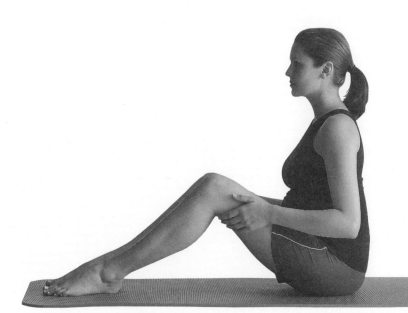

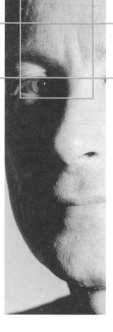

authors' introduction

Yolande and I have helped many pregnant women through the exciting and rewarding experience of improving the body's posture and increasing its strength and flexibility during pregnancy. We have shared their excitement as well as their fears and worries about exercising while pregnant. We've also tried to help them find a path between the truths and myths presented to them by well-meaning friends and family.

Twenty-two years ago I came across Pilates as a dancer at the London School of Contemporary Dance. Though it was part of our daily training, I didn't really understand the importance of it. It wasn't until I began practising Pilates to repair a back injury that I really began to appreciate its power and effectiveness. I loved what it did to heal my body.

It is so exciting to see the recent boom in popularity that Pilates has enjoyed. From both the experience of my own back injury and my extensive work within the fitness world, I have come to appreciate the true value and significance of the technique.

My goal is to pass on the knowledge that I have acquired over the years and to share the secrets I've found that make this work successful. Pilates is a very varied technique, and it can be taught in many formats and styles. Thus it lends itself particularly well to adaptation for both the pregnant and the postnatal woman, offering a safe and rewarding exercise regime.

During my past 20 years as a Pilates instructor, I have had the opportunity to work with many pregnant women, helping each one to find the level that is right for her, keeping comfort and safety a priority by using pregnancy modifications that are an essential part of the programme. In this book, we take into consideration how a woman's body changes during each trimester of pregnancy and offer modifications to suit varying levels of fitness at each stage.

Understanding the Pilates principles is crucial to gaining the maximum benefit from the movements, particularly of those working with the transverses abdominis and pelvic floor – the core muscles involved in pregnancy and childbirth. As Pilates focuses on posture, and the body and posture change so much during pregnancy, Pilates is a gentle form of exercise that naturally meets the needs of pregnant women.

No one series of exercises suits all pregnant women because each woman's experience of pregnancy is so individual. Back pain and issues with posture in pregnancy, for example, are often related to specific problems that were experienced before pregnancy and can be improved through movements focusing on these areas. In this way, the book helps women work on issues related to their particular experience of pregnancy, as well as underlying issues that may need to be dealt with after childbirth.

Performing the movements and techniques will prove to be a valuable and crucial part of your pregnancy – helping you keep fit, prepare for childbirth, and – as experience has shown us – recover more quickly, enabling you to return to a normal and active life afterwards. I hope *Pilates for Pregnancy* helps you on your own exciting journey to health and fitness in pregnancy and beyond childbirth.

This book would not be possible without the valuable contribution of Yolande Green, whose knowledge and drive has enhanced our work with pregnant clients. My immense thanks

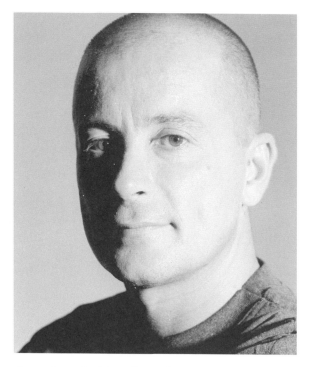

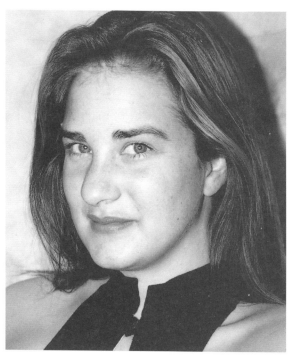

also to those who have influenced my teaching, helped me to develop different skills and shown me that there is no single way to teach Pilates.

Over the years, Yolande and I have worked with many women during and after pregnancy, and we have always found the Pilates training not only to be one of the most beneficial types of exercise to do during pregnancy, but also, for many, the most essential.

Most people will tell you that prevention is better than cure. By working safely and effectively during your pregnancy, you can assist in reducing the sometimes frequent painsd and problems associated with pregnancy. For some people, these symptoms do not become troublesome until years after the pregnancy, but a weakness (in the back, for example), however small, may become exacerbated by the ongoing demands of daily life.

With this book, Yolande and I hope that you will be able to develop a programme to help keep you strong and healthy throughout all the stages of your pregnancy and well into your postnatal recovery. We also believe that, once you have experienced the benefits of Pilates during pregnancy, you will want to continue your programme as part of your daily life, for many years to come.

Michael's profile

With more than 24 years of experience in Pilates, Michael first started working with the Pilates technique while he was a dancer at the London School of Contemporary Dance. He trained with Alan Herdman, the first teacher to bring Pilates to the United Kingdom from the United States. In 1982, he opened his own studio, Body Control, in London's Covent Garden.

Two years later, Michael moved to Texas, running a studio for the Houston Ballet Company while training in the new Fonda-established aerobics. Michael is the company director of the Pilates Institute, the United Kingdom's leading Pilates training company. He has choreographed many successful shows, including *The Blues Brothers*, Argentine's *My Fair Lady* and *Godspell*.

Yolande's profile

Yolande has been an instructor in the fitness industry for more than 11 years, teaching aerobics, step, spinning, body conditioning and Pilates. She is currently studying for an M.Sc. in health and fitness while researching exercise during pregnancy. She has worked in maternity hospitals and physiotherapy departments, including the Portland hospital in London, and is involved in the GP referral scheme, working with special populations.

Yolande is the company director of the Schools' Fitness Advisory Service, a training company for exercise teachers in secondary schools and also serves as a presenter and tutor for the Pilates Institute. She has run many successful pre- and post-natal exercise and education groups, and has given presentations at fitness conventions and workshops around the world.

what is pilates?

In recent years, there has been a renewed interest in exercise techniques that acknowledge the power of the mind. Pilates, like Feldenkrais, the Alexander technique and yoga, falls under this mind–body umbrella. All these techniques offer alternative philosophies to conventional thinking about health and fitness. Pilates is a technique that approaches the fitness of the body as a whole, working to improve strength, mobility and alignment.

Mind and movement

Pilates is named after its inventor, Joseph Pilates, who formulated the exercises in the 1920s. There are 34 original Pilates movements. As well as matwork, there are also equipment-based routines. These pieces of equipment, devised by Joseph Pilates himself, have strange and wonderful names such as The Wunda Chair, The Cadillac and the Pedi-Pul. In a traditional Pilates studio, half of the session is worked on the equipment, while the other half performed in matwork exercises. Each one offers different benefits.

The original Pilates programme consisted of 34 moves, done back to back with no modification or variation, making no allowances for an individual's needs, such as pregnancy. Our modifications to the original movements are essential, and take into consideration the many physical changes that occur during pregnancy. Although our approach is unique, there are other approaches to Pilates,

which are equally valuable to the pregnant woman.

The best way to work with Pilates is with a personal trainer, one on one. However, trainers can be difficult to find and very expensive. The goal of this book is to make Pilates accessible, so that pregnant women can educate themselves.

Joseph Pilates developed his technique from instinct, from what felt good with his own body. He changed the moves from day to day with different people that he met, according to their personal needs. The basic principles of the technique (see page 26–29) remained the same, however.

The mind is a very powerful tool. The movements that are the most challenging are usually the ones that are the least liked, but that do the most good. If a movement is easy, it indicates that there is strength or mobility in that area of the body. Use these movements as an exploration of your body and the wonderful changes that will happen during pregnancy.

They may highlight particular issues of which you may need to take note.

Core muscles

Pilates is essentially a combination of t'ai chi and yoga. The quality of movement of Pilates is very similar to t'ai chi, and many of the positions in Pilates are influenced by yoga. What makes Pilates different from both, however, is the focus on the body's centre or 'core strength'. Core strength emanates from the muscles that lie from the pelvis into the rib cage and diaphragm. These muscles work to maintain posture and support the spinal column and pelvis.

The main muscles that make up this core are the transversus abdominis (TA), multifidus, pelvic floor muscles, rectus abdominis and the obliques. The TA, as we refer to the transverse abdominis, acts as a thick corset around your centre. Imagine a tree trunk that has been cut in half. The rings of the tree represent the layers of your core strength. The TA muscle,

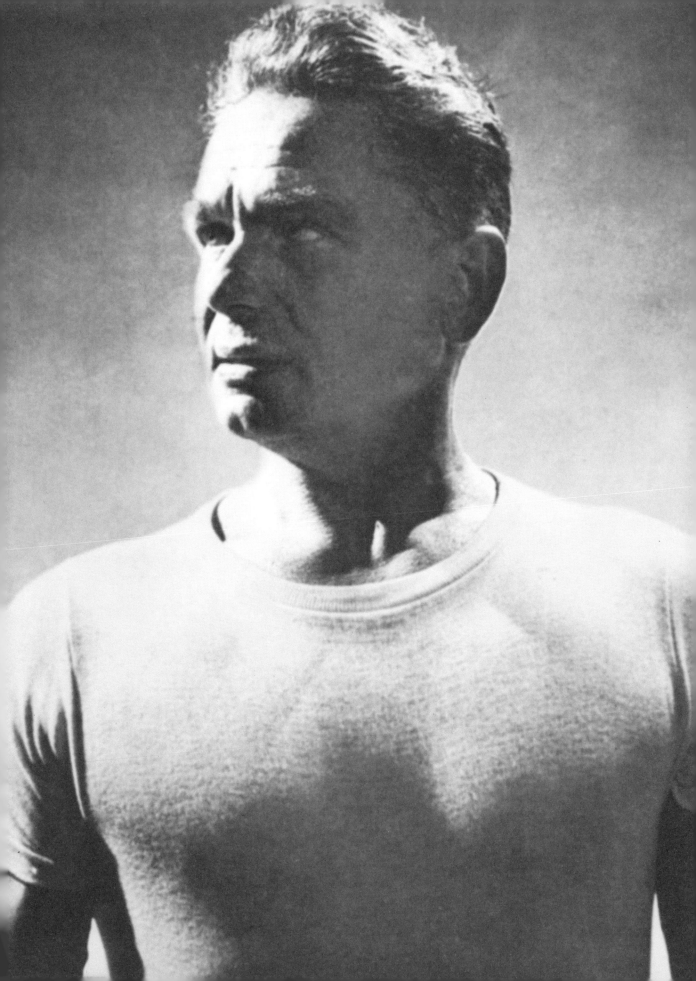

sometimes referred to as the belt muscles, is the innermost ring. It offers stability to the torso and support to your centre to help maintain a correct upright position.

All movements of the body activate the core muscles, so even when you lift your arm, muscles in your back and abdominals activate to assist this move.

During pregnancy, your core requires greater stabilization due to the changes in your posture, weight and centre of balance. Creating strength in your core muscles, TA, pelvic floor and multifidus will help to reduce some of the excessive pressure on surrounding joints, muscles and bones.

In Pilates we concentrate more on the deeper core muscles. Pilates uses a sequence of exercises to work these deep core muscles, by adding the challenge of weight to the core (lifting your leg), by adding balance (standing on one leg while maintaining neutral), or by adding movement (circling the leg). Your core is also stabilized by another group of muscles, the pelvic floor, which assist in stabilizing the pelvis and spine.

As your pregnancy progresses the muscles that make up your core (abdominal muscles and back muscles), plus the muscles that help to support you, your frame, and the weight of the growing baby become stressed and extremely challenged. During and after pregnancy, therefore, there is a great need to strengthen and retrain these areas.

Most people think of a sit-up when they think of exercising the abdominal muscles. In a sit-up most of the focus is on the rectus abdominis. As you will see later in this book these muscles lose some of their strength during pregnancy due to separation (see pages 18-19) and can become hard to train correctly during pregnancy. The deep core muscles play a very important role during pregnancy and also in assisting recovery from child birth.

Research has shown that the TA and the pelvic floor muscles are connected. When contracting the TA muscle the pelvic floor muscles also become activated. It is important to remember this connection when working through the exercises later in the book.

It is crucial that these muscles are activated before movement occurs in order to offer support and strength to the core. However because of the connection between these two muscle groups it is important that only one muscle groups is focused on at a time. For example it is not recommended that you contract the TA muscle (draw in the lower abdominals) and the pelvic floor at the same time, because one will contradict the other. This is discussed in more detail later in the book.

Beauty and benefit

Pilates has been around for the past 70 years, but has recently drawn much media coverage. Many Hollywood stars have given the technique their endorsement. As a result of such public praise, Pilates is no longer the exclusive preserve of the rich and famous. What once might have seemed like a strange cult activity is now a popular class in health clubs the world over. While some people become interested in Pilates for its cosmetic body-sculpting effects, others come to it through referrals by their medical practitioner or physiotherapist. Pilates is an excellent preventative technique that strengthens the body against potential injury.

As people with fast-changing and stressful lifestyles, we are naturally drawn to mind–body techniques such as yoga. Each technique offers us a different focus, which can be beneficial to different needs. Many practices such as yoga work on posture and holding the postural positions. T'ai chi, on the other hand, focuses on the movement quality.

Working step by step, you can change the way your body looks, moves and feels. The idea of this book is to take you through the major changes to your body during pregnancy, looking at how these changes will affect your posture, body composition and strength. Using this knowledge, we then take you through a step-by-step programme, allowing you the flexibility to adapt the exercises where necessary and to mix and match the exercises according to your body's needs.

People often ask how many times a week they should perform the exercises, and the answer is always the same: the more you do, the better you will become. Obviously, you do not want to fatigue your muscles, especially not the core muscles, as these are used in practically every activity in your normal daily routine. The key, however, is to find a balance between the two. The normally recommend guidelines are 20-30 minutes three to five times a week. Remember, Pilates is not only about the moves shown in this book, but also about paying attention to how you move and use your body throughout the day. Most of the basic exercises, such as breathing, pelvic floor exercises and connecting with your TA, can be done virtually any time and in any location.

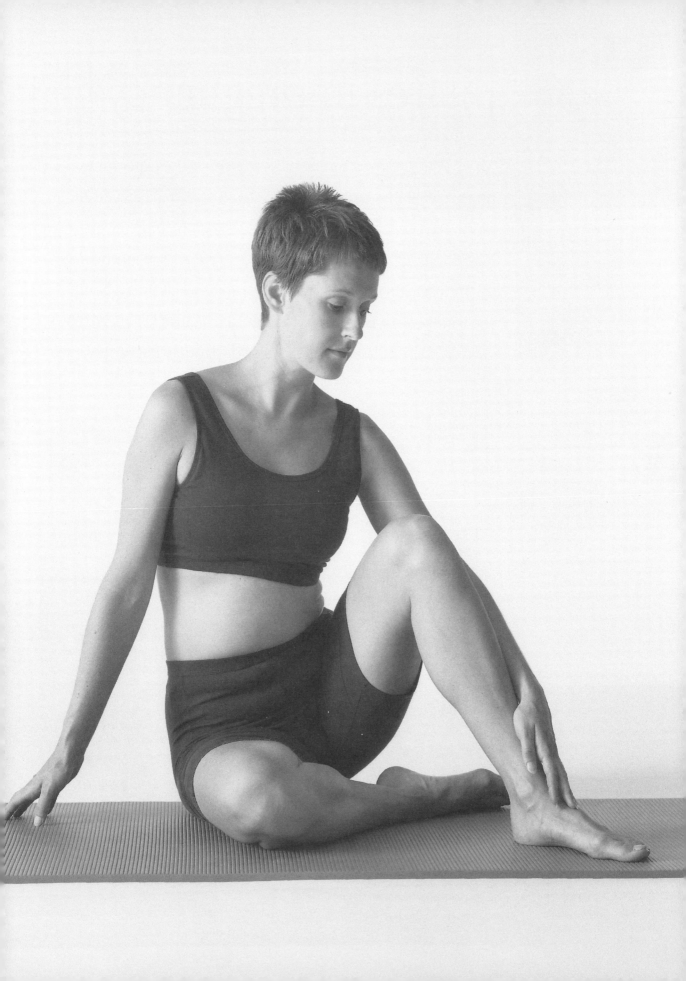

pilates in pregnancy

Many Pilates moves can be used to benefit the expectant mother, enabling her to maintain good posture, alleviate some of the recurrent aches and pains, and become more aware of her changing body. The technique also allows the mother to follow a safe and effective exercise programme throughout the whole pregnancy, one which can be adapted to meet the current stage of her pregnancy and day-to-day energy levels.

Pilates for Pregnancy takes the original Pilates exercises and movements, modifying them as necessary for each stage of pregnancy. The focus is put upon postural changes, muscle training and physical training in preparation for childbirth.

There are thousands of moves that you can call Pilates moves. Most are based on the original 34 movements, but all will apply the same eight basic principles (these are explained in greater detail on pp. 26–29). Unlike other types of exercise, you can start with Pilates at any stage of your pregnancy and still reap tremendous benefits. It also doesn't matter if you haven't trained with Pilates before. It is absolutely never too late to learn.

For many pregnant women, this is a time that they feel the greatest need and motivation to get fit and look after themselves. But you may be restricted with exercise choice in terms of what it is safe for you to do while pregnant and, even within that, what you feel physically able to do as your baby grows larger. Or you may have injuries or medical issues which restrict what exercises you are able to do; remember, these will almost certainly be exaggerated by the pregnancy.

If you have been following a Pilates programme before becoming pregnant, you may already have a reasonable amount of core strength. Don't forget that you will need to make adaptations to your current programme to take into account the changes in your body. Working through the levels, you can still create a positive, constructive and functional programme that can also be carried on postnatally, encouraging a quick recovery from childbirth.

Lying on your back during pregnancy

You can continue to lie on your back during pregnancy until it starts to feel uncomfortable. This will normally be in the middle of the second trimester; however, it may be sooner or later than this. You may also find that your breasts start to feel uncomfortable

A cautionary note

It is particularly important that you do not begin an exercise regime without approval from your doctor if you have any of the following conditions or symptoms:

- You have any type of heart or lung condition.
- You have diabetes that developed before or during your pregnancy.
- You have high blood pressure.
- You have a history of premature labour.
- Your placenta is implanted completely over or near your cervix (placenta previa).
- You suffer from physical impairments or diseases of the muscles or bones.
- You have had three or more miscarriages.
- You have experienced cramping, spotting or bleeding during this pregnancy.
- You are carrying more than one baby.

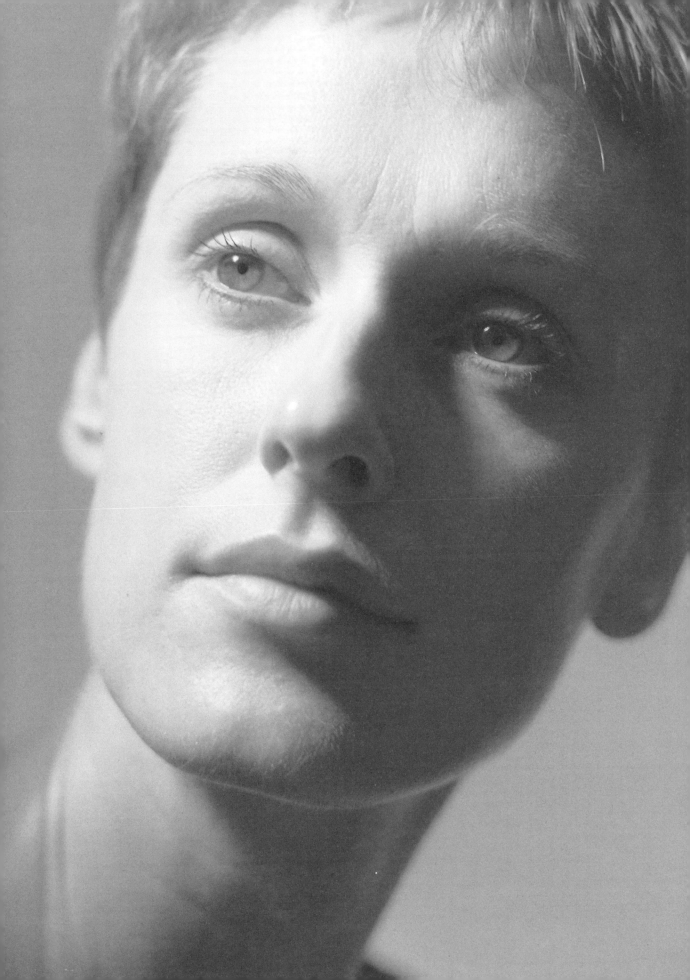

lying on them from early on in the pregnancy. Again, work with what is comfortable for you, and remember that we have already included modifications in the exercises to make allowances for these factors.

There is always great concern about lying on your back during pregnancy. This arises from that fact that you could suffer supine hypotensive syndrome, where the weight of the baby lies on the vena cava, preventing the normal circulation of blood back to the heart. This could lead to a lack of oxygen in your blood system, which in turn affects your baby's blood supply. The long-term results are that the baby may suffer from a lack of oxygen which could cause lasting damage to the baby.

To be on the safe side, we recommend that you never spend more than 5 minutes lying on your back at any one time. If you do feel dizzy during a movement, roll onto your side and rest. If symptoms continue, contact your doctor.

Exercising caution

It is vital to remember that no single exercise programme is suitable for all pregnant women. Your personal fitness level, medical conditions and exercise history will all influence your ability to perform some of the exercises.

Guidelines for safe exercise

In addition to your doctor's advice, following these general guidelines can help to keep exercise during your pregnancy safe and enjoyable. Remember, if you had an injury or problem before your pregnancy, it will still be a factor during your pregnancy, and may well be exaggerated by the pregnancy.

• Exercise at regular intervals, plan ahead and give yourself specific times to dedicate to your Pilates programme. You can't make up for lost time, so don't pressure yourself too hard to catch up.

• Always stop if you feel pain, and remember to choose the correct level for you, and reduce the levels if you need to. Stop and rest if the exercise feels in any way uncomfortable. Some exercise may just not be suitable for you. If pain persists or is severe, check with your doctor immediately.

• Do not exercise for at least an hour after eating. Exercising too soon after a meal can cause burping and abdominal discomfort. Exercising on an empty, rumbling stomach, on the other hand, may cause you to become dizzy and light-headed during the exercises.

• Don't become overheated, and avoid exercising in a hot room. You may find that you feel hotter more quickly than you did before you were pregnant. This is because the fetal temperature is 0.5 degrees centigrade higher than yours. Hormonal changes and an increase in blood supply to the skin will also contribute to your 'feeling hot'.

• If you are doing any cardiovascular work in addition to Pilates, be careful not to raise your heart rate too high. Remember that the baby's heart rate is already faster than your own.

• Stop exercising if you develop symptoms of overexertion. These include nausea, vomiting, headaches, light-headedness, dizziness, extreme shortness of breath, tightness in the chest and extreme perspiration. If any of these symptoms occur, stop exercising immediately and call your doctor.

• Exercise gently and respect your body. Always warm up slowly and avoid strain on any of your joints, especially the spine (see the warm-up section on pages 44–51).

• Sit up and lie down slowly. This is important in order to avoid straining your back. When raising or lowering your body, roll over to one side first, and use your arms and legs to assist you. You may also have slightly higher or lower blood pressure than normal, and this may make you feel a little dizzy if you change direction or position too quickly.

• Never lift both legs off the floor at the same time. This puts too much strain on the lower back muscles. Even if you were able to do this in Pilates before becoming pregnant, we suggest that you avoid exercises that require this until at least six months after you have given birth.

• You may feel an added flexibility and suppleness during pregnancy, which is due to the presence of a hormone called relaxin (see page 20), which softens the ligaments (which join bone to bone) and can cause the joints to become slightly unstable. Always make sure that you pay extra attention to your alignment when carrying out every exercise.

• Wear suitable clothing that is comfortable, supportive (i.e. support bras) and allows perspiration to evaporate as you exercise.

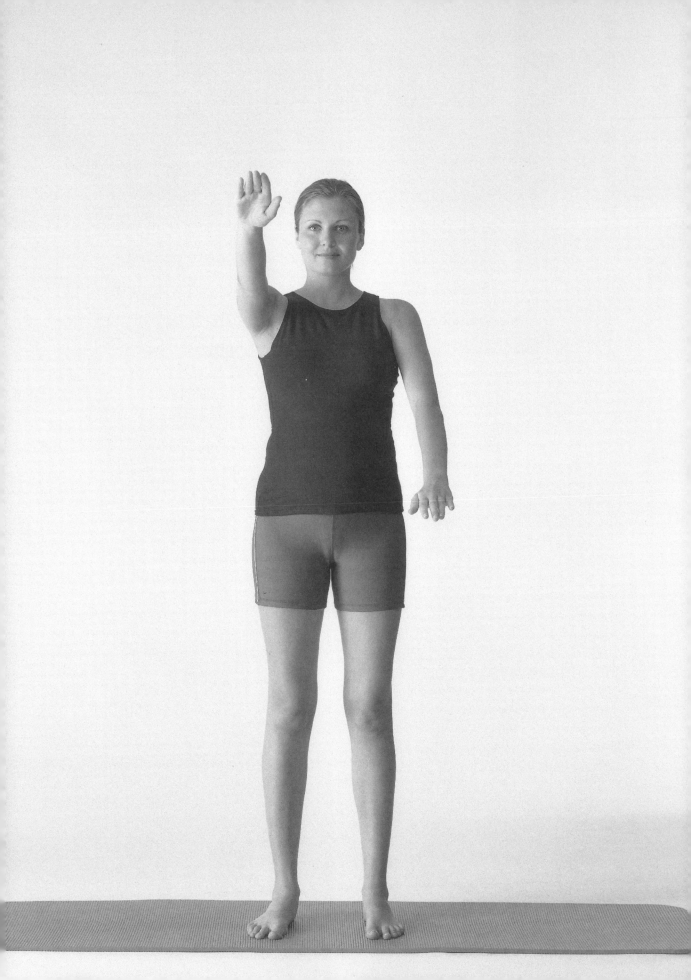

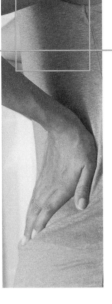

the benefits

During pregnacy, a woman's posture changes dramatically in response to the growing baby, which can cause discompfort and misalignment in different parts of her body. This may result in decreased energy levels, aches and pains, breathlessness and muscle tightness. By following a Pilates exercise programme throughout pregnancy, the mother can alleviate all these symptoms, as well as prepare for labour.

Many women suffer from back pain and other minor aches and pains during pregnancy, often until well after the baby is born. Such physical discomfort is not unusual and can sap strength, as well as interfere with sleep or rest. By paying particular attention to posture, muscular strength and balance throughout the pregnancy – and by learning how to stand, sit and move – such aches and pains can be significantly reduced or avoided altogether. For example, maintaining a good posture from the early stages can improve a woman's energy levels as her body changes. Similarly, maintaining a 'neutral alignment' of the body (see pages 32–3 for a full explanation of a neutral body position) can help relieve stress and strain on muscles, joints and ligaments that might otherwise prevent relaxation and good sleep.

Pilates exercises offer both mental and physical training. They differ from other fitness techniques by targeting the deep postural muscles, building strength from the inside out, developing core stability, re-balancing the body and bringing it into correct postural alignment.

Pilates works to develop balance, centering (keeping weight centred evenly through the joints), good posture, and abdominal and back strength, as well as working the diaphragm muscles. Pilates exercises provide an ideal preparation for the body before labour and play an important role in the body's recovery after labour. Practicing Pilates on a regular basis:

• Increases abdominal strength, thus providing support for the weight of the uterus and baby, and acting as a splint for the spine (by helping to keep it in a neutral position).

• Aids childbirth by making the pelvic floor muscles stronger and giving the mother greater body awareness so that she can focus on this area.

• Increases stamina

• Creates stronger, toned abdominal muscles that are less likely to separate severely. Also, in stronger abdominals, if separation occurs, muscles will realign more quickly. Severe separation means less support for the spine and probable back pain

• Promotes good posture and strong core strength, which help to control the amount of pelvic tilt. Excessive pelvic tilt can create posture problems and lower back pain

• Aids relaxation, improves sleep and increases energy levels

• Improves circulation and helps to prevent varicose veins and leg cramps

• Reduces general aches and pains by improving posture

• Aids breathing in labour and reduces shortness of breath during pregnancy

• Quickens postnatal recovery

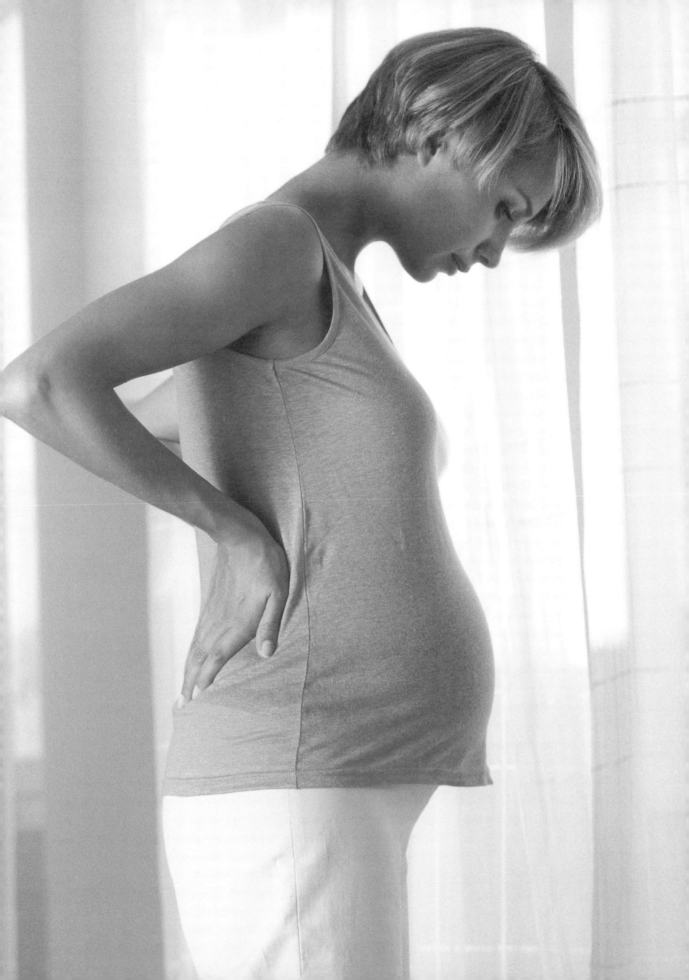

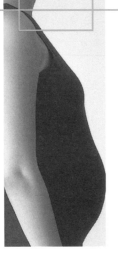

posture in pregnancy

Posture is maintained by a subconscious mechanism known as the postural reflex. This reflex can be positively influenced by exercise and can help lead to improvements in body awareness. Pregnancy can have many negative effects on a woman's posture, some of which remain with the mother postnatally and into subsequent pregnancies. The Pilates technique will help you become aware of these changes in your posture.

During pregnancy, the pelvic tilt affects the curve of the lumbar spine. This is because the sacrum (the lower part of the spine) and coccyx (tailbone) are attached between the two hip bones that form the pelvis. Muscles in the abdominals, especially the transversus abdominis, are essential for the maintenance of a correct pelvic tilt. As the uterus and baby grow and the weight increases, the abdominal muscles have to work harder to maintain this position.

Unfortunately, many women lack the abdominal strength to support the weight of the growing uterus and baby, and maintain a correct pelvic tilt. This causes the back to overcompensate by increasing the lumbar curve, which in turn increases the forward tilt of the pelvis – resulting in painful lower back pain. Additionally, the abdominal muscles become stretched due to the expanding size of the uterus and as a result offer less support for the spine.

Many pregnant women also experience shoulder and upper back aches as the breasts grow. The increased weight of the breasts causes the shoulders to start to roll forwards, resulting in the muscles of the chest becoming tight and the muscles in the back becoming stretched.

Pregnancy is a very challenging time for a woman to concentrate on her posture. Month to month, especially in the last trimester, changes in her centre of gravity and alignment occur continually. This means that she needs to re-educate her body on a regular basis as to what is 'neutral alignment'.

Standing

When you are standing, be aware of the tendency to relax your abdominal muscles and arch your back to compensate for the weight of the uterus. The following technique will help you to prevent arching of your lower back and tightness in the upper back and shoulders.

Tuck in your chin slightly to align your head with your body. Tip your tailbone down slightly. Imagine that

Top-to-toe body check

Try to do this basic posture check at least once a day. As the day goes on, you may find you become tired and less aware of your posture, so this quick body check will help you maintain a neutral posture.

- Raise your eyes slightly as if looking over the horizon.
- Draw your shoulders gently down and away from the ears.
- Roll the shoulders slightly back, opening the chest.
- Now roll the pelvis forwards and back until you feel that it is in an upright position and that there is little tightness in your lower spine
- Make sure that your feet are hip-width apart, with your toes very slightly turned out.
- Check that the knees are following the line of your feet, and not rolling in or out.
- Find the point in your feet where your weight is evenly distributed.
- Slowly breathe in and out, inhaling through the nose and exhaling through your mouth.

you have a long tail hanging down between your legs. As you tilt your tailbone, the tail drops further between your legs. Stand with your feet just slightly wider than your hips, with feet facing forwards. Keep your knees slightly bent. Concentrate on centring your weight through the centre of your hips, knees and feet. Draw your shoulders away from your ears, then allow them to drop slightly back. You will feel your chest open and the tightness in your neck and shoulders dissipate.

If you have to stand for a long period of time, try placing one foot up on a low stool or step to help prevent your pelvis from tipping forwards. If this is not possible and you have to stand for a long time on both feet, shift your weight from one foot to the other or rock back and forth from your heels to your toes.

Exercising the muscles in your legs will help to force blood back up your legs, helping to prevent swelling and varicose veins.

Sitting

You also need to maintain correct alignment when sitting, especially if you are sitting for long periods of time.

Sit straight up in the chair. Tilt your pelvis and gently hollow your lower abdominal muscles (transversus abdominis). Then slide your buttocks slightly forwards from the back of the chair so that your lower back comes into contact with the chair back.

If you need to lean forwards, to type or write at a desk, push your buttocks against the back of the chair and lean your body forwards while keeping your transversus abdominis (TA) hollowed. It may also be helpful while sitting to raise your feet on a low stool.

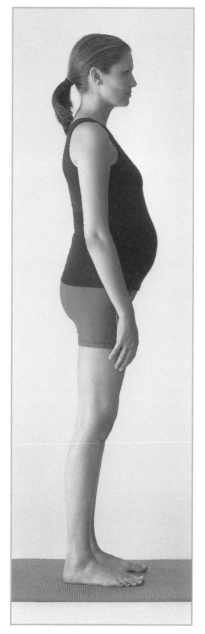

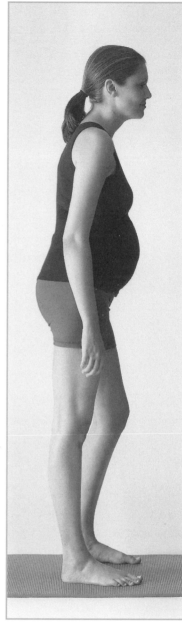

Good posture
The feet are hip-width apart, weight is distributed evenly through both feet and the pelvis is in neutral (not excessively rolled forwards or back). The spine is in neutral, alleviating compression in the lower spine, the chest is open, the shoulders are rolled slightly back and down, and the neck is lengthened.

Bad posture
The weight is unevenly distributed – most of the weight is over the right hip and ankle. Hips are shifted forwards and to one side, causing an imbalance. The abdominals are forward, placing strain on the lower back and pelvis. The shoulders are rolled forwards, causing strain to upper back muscles; the neck is short and compressed; and the head is extended forwards.

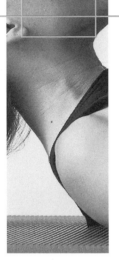

ligaments and separation

One of the biggest changes to a woman's body during pregnancy is to the ligaments and fibrous tissue. The body cleverly adapts to the growing baby by making minor changes to its structure. By being aware of these changes and exercising caution when needed, these changes should not have any long-term effects on the mother's body, allowing her to recover after labour without any added injuries or imbalances.

During pregnancy, the body produces a hormone called relaxin. It is produced around the second week of pregnancy and reaches its highest level by the end of the first trimester. It then drops by approximately 20% and remains at that level until after the birth. The role of relaxin is to relax the ligaments of the pelvis and allow separation of the joint surfaces, allowing more space within the pelvis to accommodate the growing baby and prepare for labour.

Unfortunately, relaxin is not confined to just the pelvic area; it can affect fibrous tissue anywhere in the body such as the hips, knees, elbows, ankles and spine. This means that during pregnancy you may feel an increase in your flexibility; however, be careful not to take advantage of this increased flexibility, as it may cause long-term damage to the stability of your joints.

You may also experience some slight discomfort in the pelvic area, especially in front of the pelvis where

the two sides of the pelvis meet, in the lower pubic area and also in the back of the pelvis where the pelvis joins the lower part of the spine. Some exercises may help to loosen this area and relieve the pain, but be careful of any exercise which increases the level of discomfort. Seek advice from your GP if you are uncertain.

Relaxin remains in the body for three to five months after childbirth, longer for those mothers who are breastfeeding. Try to allow your body time to recover postnatally before moving on to some of the more advanced moves or exercise programmes, especially those which include high-impact work.

The round and broad ligaments

Two major ligaments, the round and broad ligaments, help to support the weight of the uterus. The round ligaments are situated on either side of the uterus and connect at the front of the pelvis (see picture 1). Sometimes during exercise you may experience

slight discomfort in the groin or vaginal area when the enlarged uterus shifts suddenly, which could be caused by the round ligament. The broad ligament (picture 1) attaches into the lumbar spine and the uterus sac. As the baby's weight increases, abdominal muscles weaken, the pelvis rolls forwards and the weight of the uterus sac can pull on the broad ligament, which in turn can cause some discomfort in the lumbar spine area. If the abdominal muscles – especially the transverses abdominis (TA) muscle – are strong, they will help to prevent the pelvis rolling too far forwards and pulling on the broad ligament.

Separation

The abdominal muscles have to stretch both in width and length to accommodate the growing uterus. As well as the muscles themselves stretching, this expansion is facilitated by the linea alba (a fibrous union connection – the two sides of the rectus abdominis, obliques and

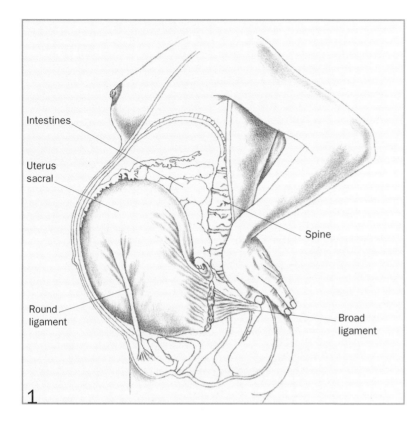

Intestines

Uterus
sacral

Spine

Round
ligament

Broad
ligament

1

1 The round and broad ligaments:
the round ligament is attached from
the uterus sacral into the front of the
pelvis; remember, these are situated
on both sides of the body. The broad
ligament extends from the uterus
into the lower part of the spine.

2 This picture shows the abdominals
in a non-pregnant woman. Notice the
alignment of the rectus abdominis.

3 Here the abdominals are seen
during the third trimester of
pregnancy. The linea alba has
lengthened and the rectus muscles
now lie further apart.

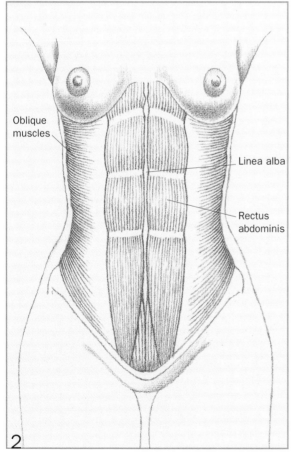

Oblique
muscles

Linea alba

Rectus
abdominis

2

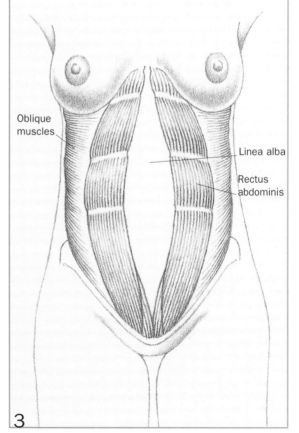

Oblique
muscles

Linea alba

Rectus
abdominis

3

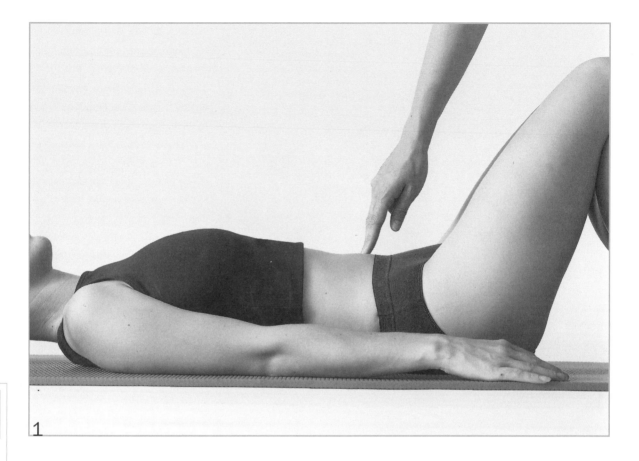

1 Lie on your back with your knees bent and feet flat. Place two fingers vertically onto the abdominals just above or below the belly button.

transversus; see picture 2 on p. 21). This condition of separation is called diastasis recti. In some cases, the rectus abdominis, which is normally side by side, may actually become separated by 3 to 6 inches. If you have previously had a baby, the muscle separation may be greater, and you may carry the baby out in front earlier.

Separation in symphysis pubis

In preparation for childbirth, the pelvis also changes form slightly. The joints that hold the bones of the pelvis together loosen and separate due to the hormone relaxin. This joint is called the symphysis pubis. It joins the

pubic bones together at the front of the pelvis. It is a thick pad of cartilage which acts as a buffer between the two bones. It also plays an important role in the stability of the pelvis. This is one of the main areas affected by relaxin during pregnancy.

This is the body's way of enlarging the space inside your pelvis to make it easier for the baby to pass through during delivery. You may actually be able feel a separation in your bones of up to an inch simply by placing a finger in the middle of bone that lies above your vagina.

The amount of separation can be affected by exercises and the strength of your abdominals. Some exercises may increase the amount of separation. These include moves when you are not able to control the doming of the lower abdominals. This is when you feel the

lower tummy muscles pushing out, for example, when lifting your head off the floor in a normal sit-up.

The TA (transverses abdominis) muscle which runs round the lower part of the abdominals links into the linea alba (the muscle that runs down the centre of your stomach). By practising the basic Pilates moves, you can help to prevent the abdominals separating too far and assist in the stability of your core (ie spine, pelvis and abdominals).

Pilates exercises which focus on the TA will also help greatly with postnatal recovery and the return of the abdominals to their normal state. Remembering to try to draw in the lower abdominals first will assist with this. These exercises can be done at any time – sitting at a desk, while out shopping, waiting for a bus etc. Try to

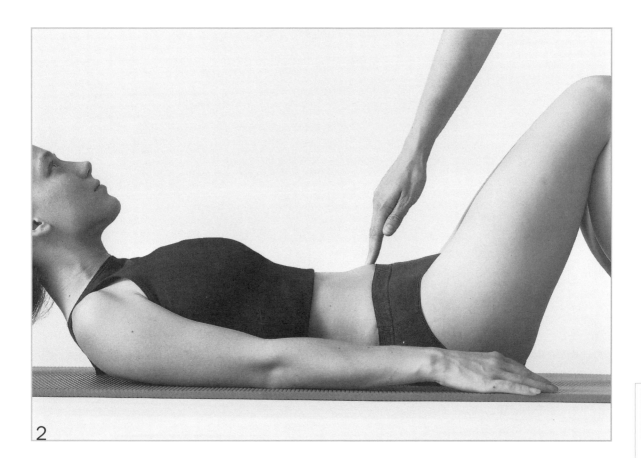

2

2 Gently lift the head and shoulders off the floor. At the same time, gently press down with the fingers, moving them side to side to find the sides of the rectus.

imagine the stomach muscles drawing in gently to hug the baby.

The separation test

Postnatally, you can test how far your abdominals have separated. This will be a good indication of how quickly your body has recovered. If this is not your first pregnancy, the muscle separation and weakness may be greater, and you may feel that you have carried the baby further out in front than in previous pregnancies. This will also apply to women carrying more than one baby. The following test should be comfortable to do a week

after childbirth. If you find it difficult to do this test by yourself, ask a friend or partner to help you.

Lie on your back with your knees bent and feet flat on the floor. Place two fingers vertically side by side above or below the belly button. Gently press the fingers down into the abdominals (this should not cause pain or discomfort), and gently lift your head and shoulders off the floor. As you lift your head, you should be able to feel the two sides of the rectus abdominis close together between your fingers. If you do not feel the sides of the rectus wall, use your fingers to measure the side of the gap – for example, can you fit two or three fingers in the gap – so that the outside fingers are touching the sides of the rectus. If the gap is two fingers or more, this means that separation is

still present. This condition is known as diastasis recti.

To allow the rectus to realign, you should avoid any exercise that requires you to lift your head, ie sit-ups, or any exercises which involve twistng in the waist, such as oblique curls. Stay with the basic Pilates exercises that focus on working through the TA as explained above.

This test can be repeated on a regular basis to help you to monitor the progress. If you feel that the rectus is failing to realign after a few months, ask your midwife or GP to check for you. If this is not your first child or you have had a multiple birth, it may take longer for the rectus to realign.

Doing sit-up style exercises too quickly may cause the rectus to remain separated permanently, causing a dome-like stomach.

the principles

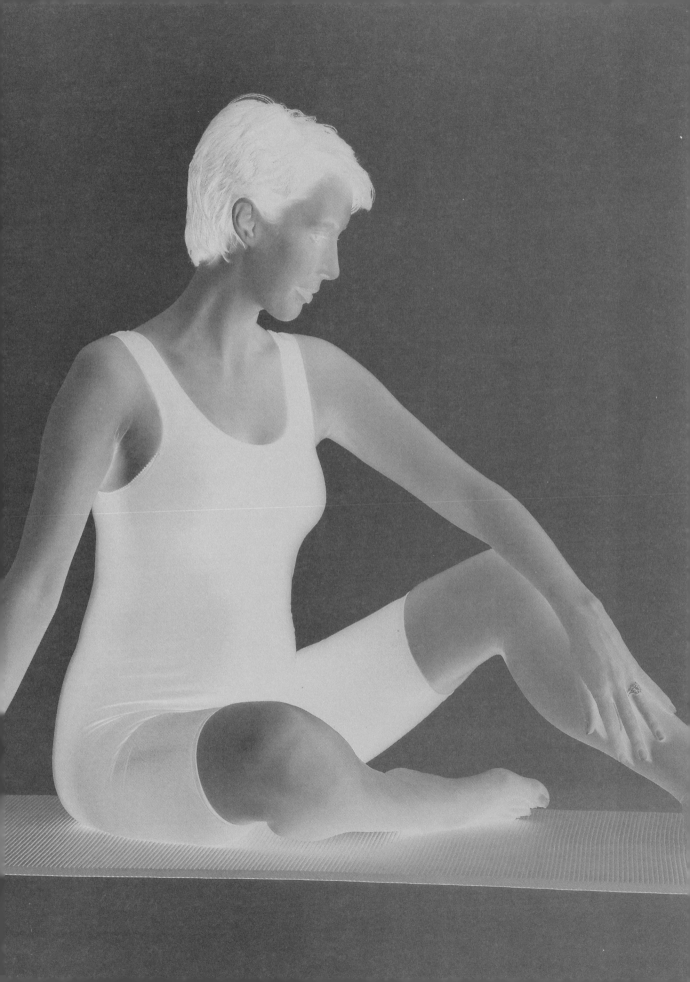

the principles

This Pilates programme targets the deep postural muscles, to build strength from within by stabilizing the torso. The body becomes realigned, the muscles balanced, and the whole body moves more efficiently. Using your mind and body together, you will develop body awareness and control. The Pilates exercises are built around eight principles: concentration, breathing, centring, control, precision, movement, isolation and routine.

Concentration

'Always keep your mind wholly concentrated on the purpose of the exercises as you perform them.'
Joseph Pilates

Controlling our thoughts, much like controlling our actions, is not as easy as it might first appear. When we are under pressure, our thoughts can become very erratic and spin off in random directions. If we are stressed, tired or feeling uncomfortable, going to sleep can be difficult, especially during the third trimester of pregnancy. This is because we are distracted and unable to 'switch off', and unwelcome thoughts pop into our heads despite our best efforts.

Your first attempts at unfamiliar movements may feel strange and awkward. It is very easy to fall into the trap of performing only the moves that you enjoy when what you need to do are the ones that you do not like. Only by concentrating can you properly control your actions.

Breathing

'Breathing is the first act of life. Our very life depends on it. Millions have never learned to master the art of correct breathing.'
Joseph Pilates

Correct breathing takes time to master. Of all the elements, this is the one most people find difficult to achieve. It is usually the last to fall into place. The main thing to remember is to breathe as frequently as you would naturally. If you find a movement is too slow for a single breath and you need to take another, then take one.

The wrong way

Whatever you do, don't hold your breath while exercising. Most people hold their breath if they pick up something heavy, much as weightlifters would when picking up a barbell. This type of breathing is called the Valsalvic method, and it results in a stressful increase in blood pressure. Keep your breathing continuous.

For exercises on mastering the breathing turn to page 34.

Centering

'Pilates develops the body uniformly, corrects wrong postures, restores physical vitality, invigorates the mind and elevates the spirit.'
Joseph Pilates

The practice of centering focuses on the rib cage, the spine and the pelvis. Pilates movements concentrate on these muscles. The difficulty lies in the fact that these are inner muscle groups. This means that unlike with the bicep muscle, which you are able to watch at work, you have to rely on the feeling of the muscles at work as opposed to seeing them actually move, as they lie beneath the surface.

Try to think of these muscles as a corset wrapped around your centre, from the rib cage right down into the pelvis. As the corset draws in, it helps to support the spine. During pregnancy, your corset may lose its

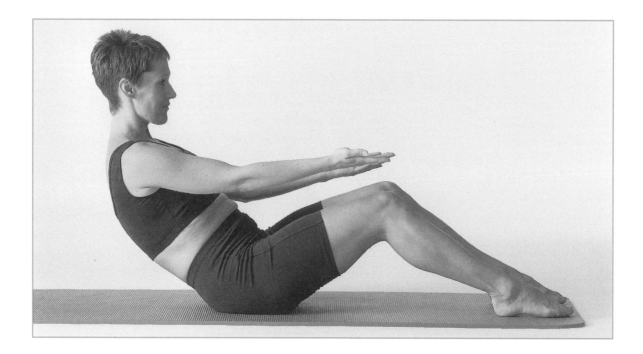

elastic! By performing centering exercises and Pilates movements, however, you can help to maintain the elasticity of these muscles.

Another way to look at these deep inner muscles is to think of your centre as a tree. If the tree were cut in half, you would be able to see many rings. The rings on the outside (the bigger ones) are the muscles that you can see in the mirror when you exercise, ie your six-pack muscles. The smaller circles towards the centre of the tree are the deep inner muscles that need to be worked; the centre of the tree is your spine. As you learn to centre and breathe (see page 34), try to draw the circles closer into the centre.

Centering is also about finding the centre of all your major joints. When standing, try to keep your weight centred through all your joints, especially your spine, pelvis and knees. This will be challenging as your pregnancy progresses, as your centre of gravity will continually change. On the other hand, your centre in your knees and spine will remain the same, although you will need to re-educate your body on finding these centres.

Control

'Good posture can be successfully acquired only when the entire mechanism of the body is under perfect control.'
Joseph Pilates

All Pilates movements are slow and controlled. They should be done at the same speed throughout. None of the actions is jerky or frenetic, putting your body at risk of injury. Slower movements are much harder to control and therefore more exacting and ultimately more effective. Practising Pilates will demonstrate both how little you previously thought about your movements and how necessary thought is to perform Pilates properly.

Precision

'The benefits of Pilates depend solely on you performing the exercises exactly according to the instructions.'
Joseph Pilates

All Pilates movements are exact and involve precise actions and precise breathing – think of synchronized swimmers and the exacting choreography that dancers can achieve. Joseph Pilates trained as both a boxer and an acrobatic circus performer. This gave him an appreciation of precision skills and an acute awareness of space and time.

Most people are unaware of the space they occupy and how their movements take place within it. Because Pilates demands that you not only move correctly but also breathe correctly, you will become more aware of how your personal space is created through the principles of precision and concentration.

Movement

'Designed to give you suppleness, grace and skill that will be unmistakably reflected in the way you walk, the way

you play and in the way you work.'
Joseph Pilates

The types of movement required for Pilates exercises are similar to those of t'ai chi, which are slow, graceful and controlled. As with t'ai chi, all Pilates movements are continuous and have no beginning and no end. Nothing is sharp, strained or forced.

No sweat

Many exercise techniques focus on repetition, requiring you to stop after each one. Pilates movements are different in that you don't pause until you have completed the required number of repetitions. Each of the movements is a long, continuous cycle, requiring greater skill to control.

Full range

It is vitally important to use your full range of movement. Check that you are working equally hard, with the same intensity and resistance, throughout your body and muscle groups. The same effort should be used to extend a muscle as to contract it. By working in this way, you will begin to develop strength and flexibility in equal measure.

Isolation

'Each muscle may cooperatively and loyally aid in the uniform development of all our muscles.'
Joseph Pilates

It is only theoretically possible to work muscles in isolation; in practice, all our muscles work together in groups. Focusing on one area develops one muscle at the expense of another. Consequently, the whole balance of the body is upset. This lopsided approach

is altogether at odds with the logic of the Pilates method.

Stamina

One of the aims of Pilates is to improve the endurance/stamina of the core muscles, challenging them to maintain strength for longer periods of time. Work on building your stamina slowly. Do not attempt the more difficult levels too soon. Pilates should be become part of your overall fitness programme, not the sole programme. Try to include some forms of aerobic work such as brisk walking.

Weak links

Try to be aware of any imbalance in muscle strength or flexibility as you perform the movements, particularly as you progress through the trimesters. Work towards the weaker of the two sets of muscles, so that balance is eventually regained. Otherwise, as you become stronger, you will remain proportionally imbalanced. Try the following exercise to help you understand this idea of balance.

Stand in a neutral position, facing a mirror. Keeping your shoulders relaxed and chest open, start an arm circle with your right arm (see page 46). Next start an arm circle with the left arm. Look at and feel the size of the circle and the movement in your shoulder and back. Compare what you feel of the muscle with what you see. Are they the same? Are both shoulders still the same height? Or is one shoulder slightly higher than the other? Try to balance the movement, reducing the arm circle of one arm to match the smaller circle of the other arm, so that both are the same. This may feel a little odd at first, but achieving this balance is vital to your Pilates programme.

Routine

'Make up your mind that you will perform your Pilates movements 10 minutes (each day) without fail.'
Joseph Pilates

The development of a routine will help you to get the most out of Pilates. It does not promise quick-fix solutions, but Pilates will help you to achieve real results by offering a gentle overhaul of your daily habits.

Making the time

The best and easiest way to make time for exercise and develop a good Pilates routine is to treat it as an important appointment, scheduling it just as you would an antenatal appointment. Devoting 30 minutes every day to the maintenance of your body is a small price indeed to pay for increased comfort and energy during pregnancy, more effective use of your muscles during labour and a quicker recovery following childbirth.

As with anything, the more you do, the more quickly you will see results. Look at your other commitments, and decide how exactly much time you can realistically dedicate to Pilates. Then be patient as you develop a regular routine.

Keeping it up

Unfortunately, fitness is not something that we can store up in our bodies. Once you stop exercising, many of the benefits you have gained will be lost. Routine is about finding a way to perform the exercises on a regular basis and trying to make this an intrinsic part of your lifestyle. The benefits you see and feel should motivate you to keep Pilates up long after your pregnancy.

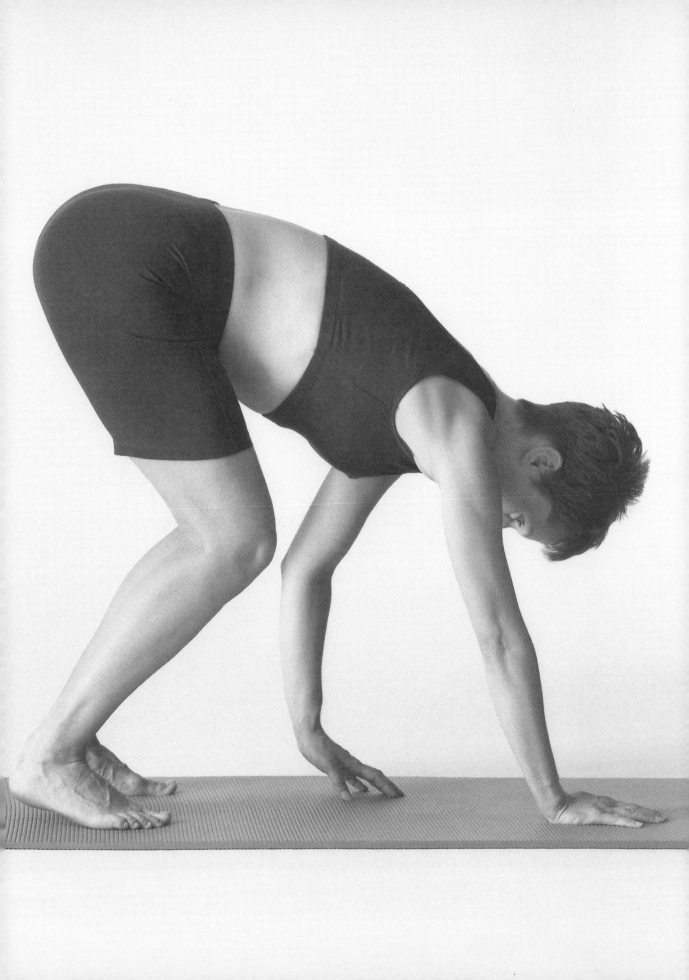

the pelvic floor

The pelvic floor or 'pelvic diaphragm' helps to support the abdominal organs and the growing uterus during pregnancy, and will stretch to assist with the birth. In particular, working with the pelvic floor muscles during pregnancy will help to make you aware of the internal muscles and your ability to activate and control them. It will assist you in relaxing these muscles during labour, facilitating childbirth.

The pelvic floor also responds to sudden rises in abdominal pressure such as during coughing, sneezing, laughing and jumping. The pelvic floor is a hammock of muscles, which passes from the pubic bones in the front of the pelvis to the coccyx, at the back of the pelvis. It fans out on either side to attach to the pelvic bones. The hammock is divided into two halves to allow room for the entryways of the urethra, vagina and anus. Try to think of your abdominal muscles and back muscles as a cylinder. The base of the cylinder is made of a fibrous stretchy material (this is the pelvic floor). The front of the cylinder is clipped, stretches across the base and is clipped on the

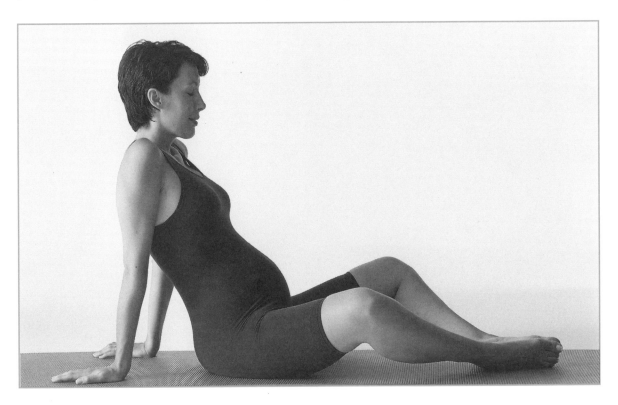

other side. As you start to fill the cylinder with baked beans (the weight of the baby), the fibrous base keeps them from falling out of the bottom. If the base is strong, it will support the weight of added beans; if not, it may struggle with any increase in weight.

Exercising the pelvic floor

If the muscle tone of your pelvic floor is strong and like a piece of new elastic, the muscle will have the ability to stretch, allowing the baby to pass through during childbirth, then return to normal afterwards. If the muscle lacks tone and strength, it may become overstretched and weak, reducing the muscle's ability to contract strongly and quickly.

During pregnancy, the relaxin (see page 20) will also affect the fibrous tissue of the pelvic floor to enable it to stretch adequately during childbirth. After childbirth, the pelvic floor muscles are stretched, weakened and bruised. Pelvic floor exercises help to tone the muscles to prevent further damage and aid recovery.

The following exercises will help you to maintain the strength and tone in your pelvic floor, as well as increase your awareness of these muscles so that you can consciously relax them during delivery of the baby. They can be done at any stage of the pregnancy.

1 Sit, stand or lie down comfortably.
2 Think about your vagina and anal area. Try to gently tighten them as if you were trying to stop the flow of urine midstream.
3 Tighten them as much as you can (like a clenched fist), we call this 100%.
4 Release them halfway, so that you are only tightening the muscle to 50%, then relax a little further, to about 30%.
5 The pelvic floor is most effectively worked at 30%, not 100%. Once you have established how to find 30%, try to hold it to a slow count of five,

breathing normally. Don't panic if you don't master this straight away, as it takes a bit of practice.

1 Relax your pelvic floor. Consider this the ground floor of the lift.
2 Draw the pelvic floor up as high as it will go, to the tenth floor.
3 Relax and begin again, this time only drawing up halfway to the fifth floor, slowly releasing to the third floor. This is your 30% range.
4 Now that you have found third floor, practise by starting on the ground floor and working up through the floors, remembering to stop to let people get in and out the lift at each floor.

In the third trimester, you will need to learn how to relax the pelvic floor as well as to contract it. Do the above exercise, but this time when you get to the ground floor, release down and into the parking lot, feeling the floor relax and open as you open the doors.

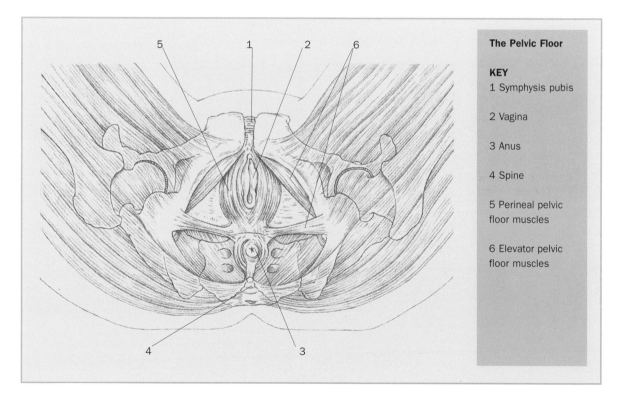

The Pelvic Floor

KEY
1 Symphysis pubis

2 Vagina

3 Anus

4 Spine

5 Perineal pelvic floor muscles

6 Elevator pelvic floor muscles

finding neutral

Neutral is a way of explaining the position of your body. To stand or lie in a neutral position means that all the joints are in neutral alignment, including the spine and the pelvis. If you exercise or even go about your daily tasks with your body constantly out of the neutral position, you run the risk of creating muscle imbalances and excessive strain upon certain joints, such as the spine.

This section is designed to help you understand how to find neutral and how to maintain a neutral position during the exercises. Once you have found neutral, the challenge in the exercise is to maintain neutral while adding movement. The following exercises will help you to find neutral. Remember that with each month of your pregnancy your body will change; your neutral position will therefore also change. The following exercises should be done as part of your warm-up every session.

Finding neutral standing

Stand with feet about hip-width apart and toes pointing forwards. If this feels uncomfortable, let them relax in their neutral position. Check that your feet and knees are not rolling in or out, and that your weight is evenly balanced through your feet.

Place your hands on your pelvis and gently roll it forward and back. As you tilt the pelvis forwards, you should feel that the curve in your lower back is accentuated. When you tilt back, you should feel your shoulders start to roll forwards. Do this gently a few times, then see if you can stop in the middle of those two movements. You should now feel a natural curve in the lower spine (with no compression or pinching) – this is the neutral position of the pelvis.

Lengthen your spine; imagine that you are balancing a book on your head and that a piece of string attached to the top of your head is gently pulling you up towards the ceiling. Try to lengthen your spine, pulling your head up and tailbone down in opposite directions from one another.

Let your shoulders drop down, stretching down and away from your ears. Then let them drop back slightly and feel your chest open a bit. Be sure that your chin is not tucked in, and remember all the while the book balancing on your head.

Quick reference

1 Align your feet and knees.

Ever changing

Remember that your body will change with each month, and these changes will be felt in your posture and muscles. Each month, work to assess your new neutral position, remembering to compensate for the growing baby and thus becoming aware of how it makes your body feel.

2 Find neutral position of the pelvis.
3 Lengthen your spine from head to tailbone.
4 Lengthen shoulders away from ears.
5 Balance the book on your head!

Exercise 1

This exercise is designed to help you understand how your body feels when you add movement after having found the neutral position.

Lying on your back in a neutral position with knees bent, place your right fingers under your lower back. Feel how much space is there. The spine may be just touching the fingers,

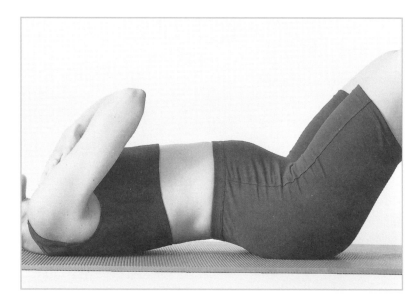

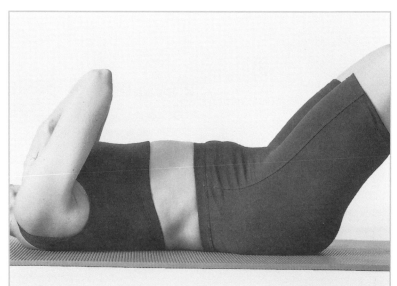

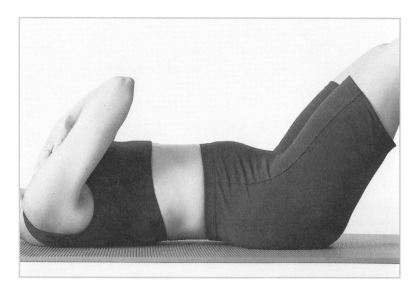

but there is no pressure on the fingers and probably not much space between the spine and the fingers. Keep your left hand on the left pelvic bone.

Stretch your right leg out to an almost straight position, then bend it back in. Did the position of the spine change? How? Try stretching the left leg out. Again, become aware of the movement in the pelvis and the lumbar spine.

If there was any movement in your hips when you lengthened either leg or when you actually changed over from the right leg to the left leg, this means that your pelvis and spine came slightly out of their neutral position.

Try the exercise again, and just become aware of the movement. Once you have found neutral again, focus on minimizing the amount of movement in the pelvis. This will activate the muscles that support the spine and pelvis to work to maintain this position. If movement does occur, it means that these muscles are not yet working sufficiently. Moving the leg challenges these muscles still further, as it makes it more difficult to hold the pelvis still. More information on how to develop control of these muscles is given later in the book.

The transversus abdominis (TA) works most effectively when the pelvis is in neutral. During pregnancy your neutral position will change through the trimesters. This is because the pelvis naturally roles forward as the uterus and baby grow out in front, thus changing the space under the lower back. Finding neutral will therefore become more challenging through your pregnancy. Develop your body awareness to find a comfortable position with minimal pressure on the lower spine.

breathing

Joseph Pilates believed in using the breath to cleanse and re-energize the body. In Pilates, we use lateral, thoracic breathing for the exercises. This means breathing into the lower ribcage and back. When breathing, always breathe in through your nose and out through your mouth. Using this technique will help you not only to control the movements and increase the flexibility of the upper body, but also to exercise the abdominal muscles:

Try the following exercise to help you understand how to breathe in.

Stand in a neutral position; place your hands on your lower ribs under the breasts. As you breathe in, feel the fingers slightly separate and the ribs expand. Then move the hands so that they are nearly under the armpits, and repeat the above.

Imagine that a friend is standing with their hands on your back, just under the shoulder blades, and try to breathe into their hands. If it helps and you are able, reach around and put the back of your hands on your back or ask a friend to stand behind you.

To help you to focus the breathing, place one hand on each side of the ribcage, one under your left breast and one under your right. Try to breathe into just the right hand only; do this in front of a mirror and check that your posture does not change as you do this, for example, by shifting your weight onto your right side. then try to breathe into just the left hand. Become aware of how your body feels from side

to side: you may feel some small differences – try to work until both sides feel the same. Try to keep your shoulders down and neck relaxed as you do this. Repeat five times and be careful not to breathe too deeply or you may start to feel dizzy.

As you breathe out, you are going to connect with your deep postural muscles in the abdominals and pelvic floor. This is called centering, as described on pages 26–7.

The following exercise should help you understand how to breathe out and to centre.

Start in a neutral standing position. Make a diamond around your belly button with your hands (see picture). Breathe in, then as you breathe out try to draw the diamond in towards the centre of your body. It's almost like a hollowing effect. Repeat the exercise, but this time focus on drawing up the pelvic floor (as covered on pages 30–1) as you breathe out.

When breathing out, either focus on the pelvic floor or the girdle – not both.

Breath control

Breathing is the first act of life. Learning to use the breath to increase control during exercise takes time and concentration. This control of breathing will help you not only with the exercises, but also with daily challenges of life such as work, stress and busy schedules.

Another way to think of it is to imagine your tummy as a brown paper bag filled with air. As you breathe out, the brown bag is gently squashed so that the size of the bag becomes smaller, and the air comes out through the top of the bag, which is your mouth!

The breathing technique does take a bit of practice, so don't panic if you don't get it right away. It certainly increases the challenge of getting all these muscles and your breathing apparatus to work in harmony.

Always breathe out while exerting the most effort in a movement.

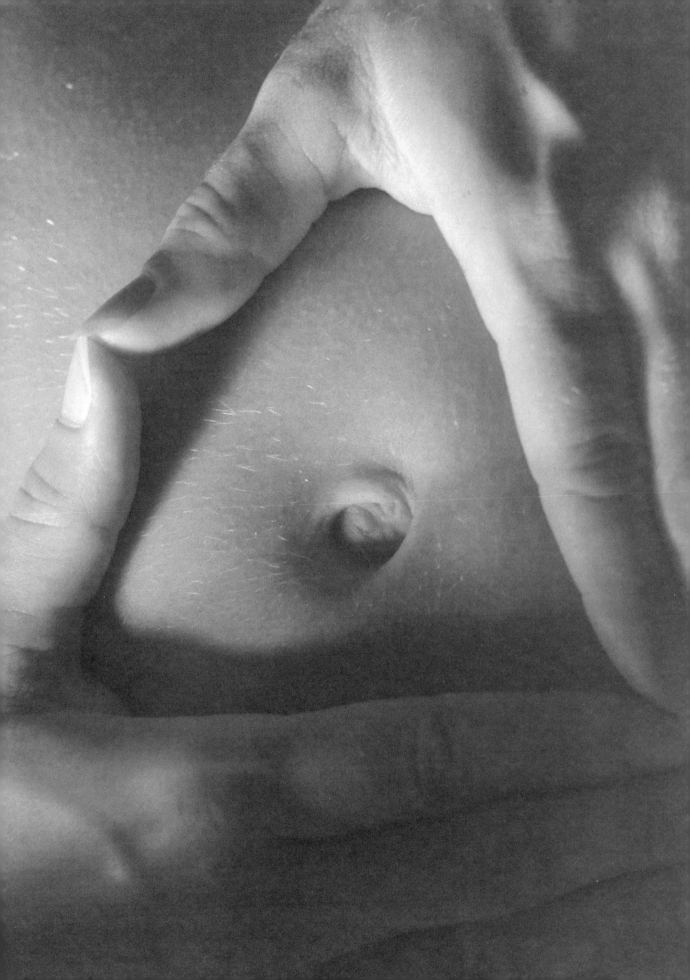

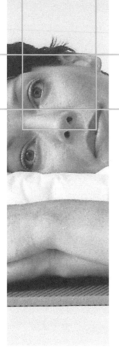

concentration and relaxation

Pilates is the 'thinking way of moving' and requires a different kind of concentration than is typically used for other exercise forms. It may not be all that important to concentrate during an aerobics class or when walking on a treadmill, but it is absolutely essential for Pilates. Concentration can be the hardest part of the exercise routine, especially when we have so many other things going on in our lives.

When working your body without engaging your mind first, you are only performing half the workout. Many times we start a new fitness regime with every good intention, but soon become bored and lacking in mental stimulation. By using visual images to engage the mind, you are able to subconsciously call upon the use of your muscles and utilize your body's movements. For example, if I asked you to lengthen your spine by imagining you are growing taller, and that an invisible cord is gently drawing yur head up towards the ceiling, not only do you use your mind to imagine this feeling, but you also use muscles you probably never knew you had.

When performing the exercises, concentrate on how your body feels as you move, breathe, lengthen and relax. Your mind is a very powerful tool and can help you achieve greater control, balance and strength.

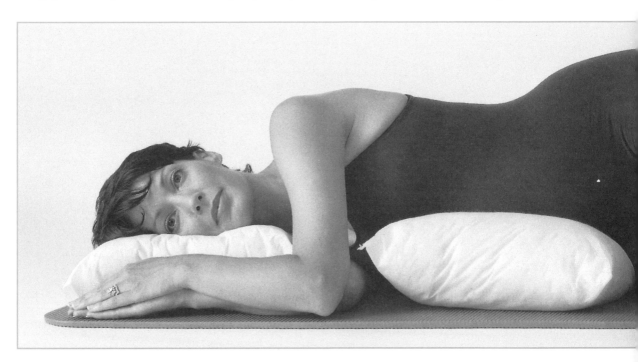

Learning to relax and focus your mind and body will help not only with the concentration, but also with your ability to relax and sleep well.

During pregnancy, many women have problems concentrating and remembering. The following exercises should help you focus. Don't panic if you forget what to do. This book acts as your reference tool day in, day out.

Exercise 1

Make sure that the space you plan to use is free of distractions. Turn off telephones and put up a 'Do not disturb' sign on your door (it's only for ten minutes!). Put on some relaxing music, but only if it has no lyrics. Otherwise you will find yourself listening to the words rather than concentrating.

Lie in a comfortable position (see picture). Give yourself plenty of cushions and support. Close your eyes and start to think about your breathing, becoming aware of how your body feels and moves as you breathe. Try to slow your breathing, making each breath longer and deeper. Remember to breathe in through your nose and out through your mouth.

As you breathe in, feel the fresh new air replenishing your body with energy and vitality. As you breathe out, imagine you are breathing out all the stale air and toxins from the depths of your lungs and body. As you continue to exhale, feel the breath going deeper into your body, starting with your abdominals, feeling your breath feeding the baby with theirs. Take this breath further into your legs, so that as you exhale you feel the breath coming up from your legs, through your tummy, chest and neck, and out your mouth.

Exercise 2

Lying in the same position, imagine that you are on a beautiful beach with the sun shining overhead and the sand warm beneath you (snuggle in a blanket if needed).

Try to listen to the waves gently lapping against the rocks and sand.

Feel the heat of the sun warming your body. Feel your feet becoming slightly heavier and gently imprinting their shape into the sand. Feel the weight of your feet against the sand, and let this feeling travel up through your legs, all the time thinking about your breathing. Feel your hips and baby gently imprinting their shape into the sand. Let the feelings travel up to your head, going slowly until the whole of your body is very gently imprinted, so that, if you were to move, the shape of your body would be left in the sand. Continue to breathe, and become aware of how your body feels and changes as you breathe and imprint.

Relaxation is an important part of any exercise programme. Learning to relax will give you a greater sense of control. If you are able to relax both mind and body it may help you to deal with the stresses and strains of daily life. It can also be used as an important tool during labour, helping you to remain calm and in control throughout.

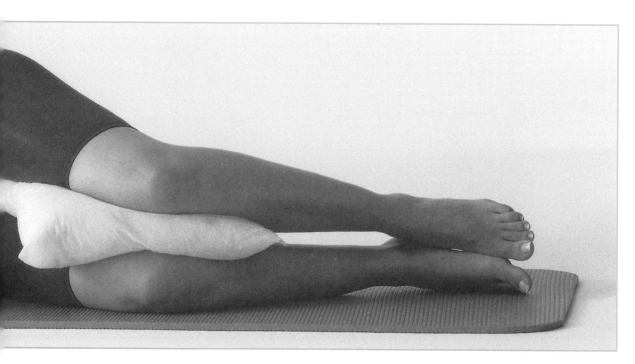

finding the right level

It is important that you work at the right level for you. This level will change as your pregnancy progresses, and it may also change from day to day depending on your energy levels and the other daily demands placed upon you. Remember, quality is far more desirable than quantity. Your body – and mind– will feel far more rewarded for the quality time and work you put in to your Pilates programme.

Pilates can be started at any stage of pregnancy; however, it is important to understand that, whatever trimester you are at, if you are new to Pilates you need to work through the basic levels first. If you are new to Pilates and in your first trimester, you may find in your second and third trimester that you can try some of the modifications. Remember, however, that it is not about achieving a workout at this stage in your life. If you are just starting with Pilates and are in your third trimester, stay with just the basic levels throughout.

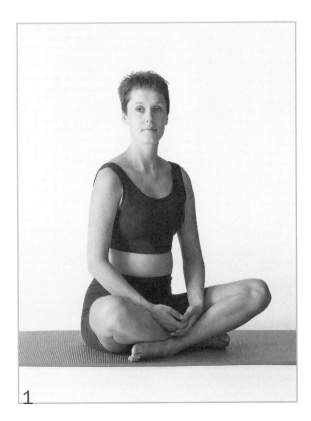

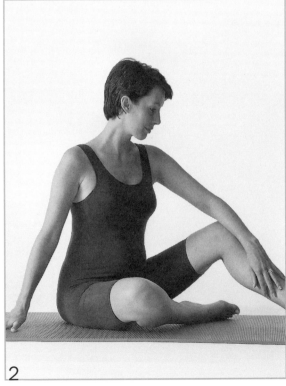

Exercising during your pregnancy is not about improving your fitness, muscle tone and strength. It is more about preparing your body for childbirth, maintaining strength and increasing your body awareness and posture. Exercise can help with the labour and help to speed up postnatal recovery. Trying to work too hard, however, can have less positive effects on your body, and it sometimes cause long term problems.

If you were not exercising before you became pregnant or have never done Pilates before, please follow the level 1 exercises. If you were doing Pilates exercises before you became pregnant and are reasonably confident with the movements, you may work through levels 2 and 3.

As your pregnancy progresses, you may need to change levels, moving down to one that feels more comfortable. If you need to stop for any reason during your pregnancy due to illness, do so without guilt. This is not a competition, and it also not about placing any extra stress on your body. When you are able to resume your routine, go back to the first level. When in doubt, always return to level one.

We have chosen three women to help represent the three different trimesters. Use these three women to help you find the right leve for you to work out. Experiment with the different levels, and learn to feel which exercise feels more comfortable and achievable for you.

We have given you guidelines for each trimester, but remember that every pregnancy is different.

How to use the charts

Follow the questions through on pages 40–1. This will help you to gain a clearer understanding of which levels to work through. If you have never done exercise or Pilates exercises before, begin with the first chart, which is level one. Follow the relevant woman to your stage of pregnancy.

The numbers are relevant to the pictures for each move. It may mean you have to flick forwards and back through the book until you become familiar with the levels, or try to copy them down or photocopy these relevant charts.

When working through the correct exercises for your trimester, if you feel the exercises are comfortable and possibly easy, try to move to the next level while still following your trimester woman. Remember, at different times in your pregnancy you may wish to switch between the levels. For example, in the first trimester, you may follow level 1; in the second trimester, you may follow Katie in the second level; and in the third trimester, follow Esther in the first level again.

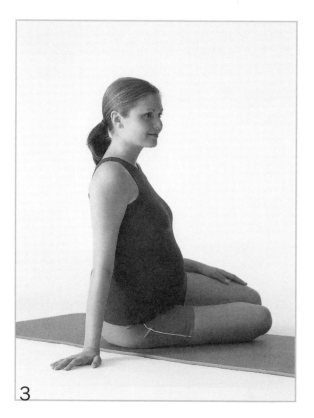

3

1 Model no. 1 is in the late stage of her first trimester of pregnancy. Because of the small risk of miscarriage in this trimester, she will be working at the first level of the exercises.

2 Model no. 2 is in her second trimester. Although she can now work a little bit harder, she varies between levels one and two of the exercises, depending on how she is feeling and how challenging she finds the exercises. She is also aware that relaxin is now an issue within her joints and that she may feel dizzy when lying on her back, which will mean she may not feel comfortable lying in this position (see pages 12–14 on safety). Remember, if you do feel dizzy at any time whilst lying on your back, simply roll over onto your side.

3 Model no. 3 is in the middle of her third trimester. She is starting to feel a little tired and occasionally breathless, so she is now working mainly at level 1. Again, she is aware of relaxin in her joints and also the concern of lying on her back (see pages 12–14).

Which level for you?

Question	Trimesters	If you answered yes	If you answered no
1 Were you exercising before you found out you were pregnant?	1st	Go to question 2	Go to question 4
	2nd	Go to question 2	Go to question 4
	3rd	Go to question 2	Work through level 1 only
2 Did you continue to exercise once you found out you were pregnant?	1st	Go to question 3	Go to question 3
	2nd	Go to question 3	Go to question 3
	3rd	Go to question 3	Go to question 3
3 Did you follow a Pilates programme before falling pregnant?	1st	Go to question 4	Go to question 4
	2nd	Go to question 4	Go to question 4
	3rd	Go to question 4	Go to question 4
4 Do you have any joint or muscle problems?	1st	Work through level 1 only	Go to question 5
	2nd	Work through level 1 only	Go to question 5
	3rd	Work through level 1 only	Go to question 5
5 Do you have any medical problems which may affect you following an exercise programme?	1st	Work through level 1 only	Go to point A
	2nd	Work through level 1 only	Go to point A
	3rd	Work through level 1 only	Go to point B

Point A – If you answered yes to questions 1, 2 and 3, and no to questions 4 and 5, then start with levels 2 and 3. Remember to change to level 1 at any time if you feel you need to.

Point B – If you answered yes to questions 1, 2 and 3, and no to questions 4 and 5, then work through levels 1 and 2.

Level one

Move	Trimester one	Trimester two	Trimester three
Push-up	1, 2, 3, 4, 5	Same	Don't do
Swimming	1, 2, 3 or 1, 4	Same	Same
Plank	1, 2	Same	Don't do
Roll-up	1, 2, 3	Same	Same
The hundred	1, 2, 3, 4	Same	Don't do
One-leg circle	1, 2, 3, 4	Same	1, 4
One-leg stretch	1, 2, 3	Same	Same
Shoulder bridge	1, 2, 3	Same	Don't do
Scissors	1, 2, 3, 4	Same	1, 2, 3, 4, or Modification
Side kick	1, 2	Same	Same
Spine stretch	Modifications 1, 2, 3	Same	Same
Spine twist	1, 2, 3, 4	1, 2, 3, 4, or Modification 1	Don't do
Double arm stretch	1, 2, 3, 4, 5	Same	8, 9, 10, 11

Level two			
Move	Trimester one	Trimester two	Trimester three
Push-up	1, 2, 3, 4, 5	Same	Don't do
Swimming	1, 2, 3 or 1, 4	Same	Same
Plank	1, 2	1, 2	Don't do
Roll-up	1, 2, 3	Same	Same
The hundred	1, 2, 3, 4	Same	Don't do
One-leg circle	1, 2, 3, 4	Same	Same
One-leg stretch	1, 2, 3	Same	Same
Shoulder bridge	1, 2, 3	Same	Don't do
Scissors	1, 2, 3, 4	Same	1, 2, 3, 4, or Modification
Side kick	1, 2	Same	Same
Spine stretch	Modifications 1, 2, 3	Same	Same
Spine twist	1, 2, 3, 4	1, 2, 3, 4, or Modification 1	1, 2, 3, 4, or Modification 1
Double arm stretch	1, 2, 3, 4, 5	1, 2, 3, 4, 5	8, 9, 10, 11

Level three			
Move	Trimester one	Trimester two	Trimester three
Push-up	1, 2, 3, 4, 5,	Same	1, 2, 3, 4, or Modification
Swimming	1, 2, 3, 4	Same	1, 2, 3 or 1, 4
Plank	1, 2	Same	Same
Roll-up	1, 2	Same	1, 2, 3
The hundred	1, 2, 3, 4	Same	Same
One-leg circle	1, 2, 3, 4, or Modification	Same	Don't do
One-leg stretch	1, 2, 3, 4, or Modification	Same	1, 2, 3
Shoulder bridge	1, 2, 3	Same	Same
Scissors	1, 2, 3, 4	Same	1, 2, 3, 4, or Modification
Side kick	1, 2, 3 or 4	1, 2, 3	1, 2
Spine stretch	1, 2, or Modification 1	Same	Modifications 1, 2, 3
Spine twist	1, 2, 3, 4	Same	1, 2, 3, 4, or Modifications 1, 2
Double arm stretch	1, 2, 3, 4, 5, 6, 7	Same	8, 9, 10, 11

the movements

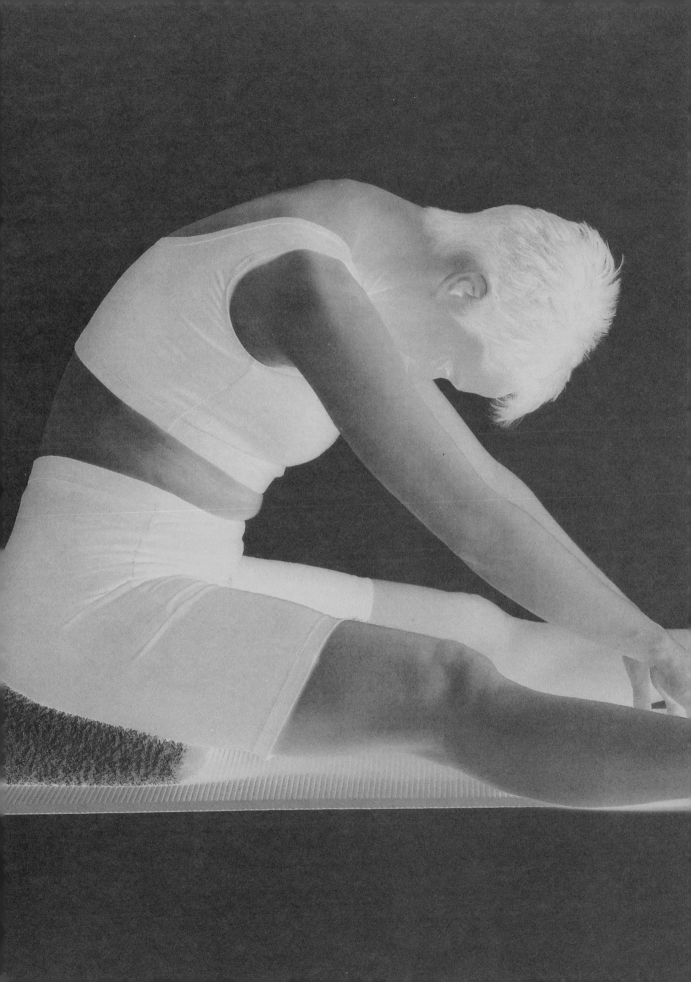

warm-ups

The purpose of the warm-up is to prepare the mind and body. The movements can be used throughout the day to stretch and relax the muscles of your back, neck and shoulders, as well as to cue you back into neutral. Begin slowly. The aim is to increase blood flow to the muscles and to mobilize the joints. Try to work each joint within a pain-free zone, making the move only as large as feels comfortable.

chest stretch

This movement helps to open out the chest and also to stretch the muscles of the chest. Try to reach a little further each time, but be careful not to arch the back as you do this; always remain in the standing neutral position. Remember to make sure that your shoulders are drawn down and away from your ears at all times.

emphasis	mobility
visual cue	'it was this big'
repeat	5–10 times

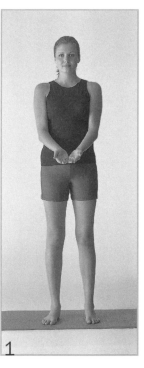

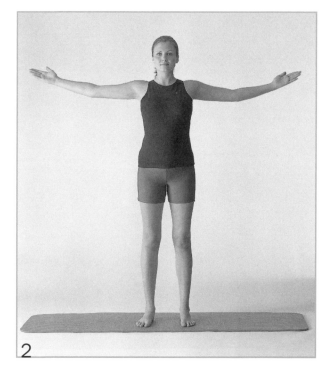

1 Stand tall with your feet about hip-width apart, knees soft and arms stretched out with palms up in front of you. Breathe in.

2 Breathe out, and stretch your arms up and to the sides. Keep your spine long by pulling that invisible string to the ceiling. As you open your arms, check that you are hollowing you lower abdominals. Do not let your back arch. Keep the movement slow and the speed constant.

swinging

This movement is suitable only in the first and second trimesters, and may become difficult due the baby's size earlier than this. Support the spine by drawing the lower abdominals in as you breathe out. The movement should be flowing and continuous, with no stop or start.

emphasis	mobility
visual cue	low bow
repeat	5–10 times

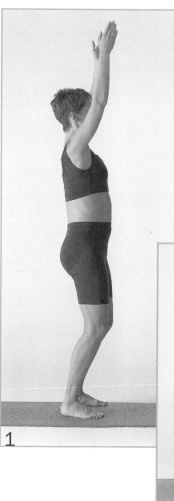

1 With your feet about hip-width apart and your knees relaxed, stretch your arms up to the ceiling – but not past your head.

2 Breathe in and let your arms fall forwards past your head. As they swing, allow your knees to bend and your back to curve. Relax your head and shoulders, and pay attention to your spine as it gently relaxes, curling over.

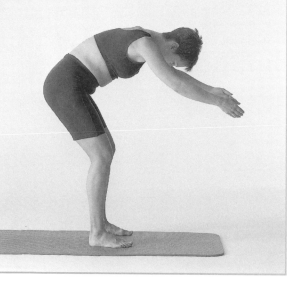

3 After reaching the curled position, breathe out, draw in the lower abdominals and slowly roll back up to the standing position. Each time you repeat the movement, try to stretch a little further towards the ceiling. Imagine a string is attached to the top of your head, pulling your entire body upwards.

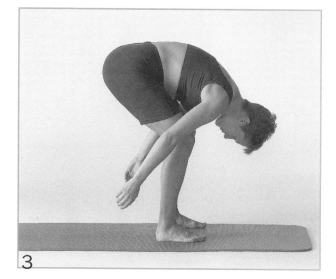

arm circles

This movement helps to mobilize your shoulders. You need to concentrate on keeping the shoulders in a line and not rotating the shoulder back as you circle. Use a mirror so that you can watch your posture. Be careful not to lean back into the move. Think about lengthening through the lower part of the spine and keeping your ribcage slightly over the pelvis. Keep your head lifted, and imagine that you are balancing a book on your head. This move can repeat in both a forward and backward direction. Remember as you breathe out to draw in and hollow your lower abdominal muscles.

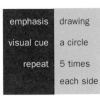

emphasis	drawing
visual cue	a circle
repeat	5 times each side

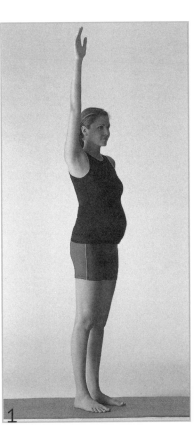

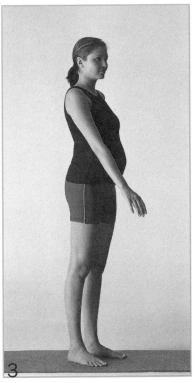

1 Stand tall with your feet apart and knees soft. Lengthen up from the top of your head to the ceiling to check that your back is correctly aligned. Keeping your right arm by your side, pressed lightly against the leg. Breathe in and lift your left arm in front of you, then lengthen to the ceiling.

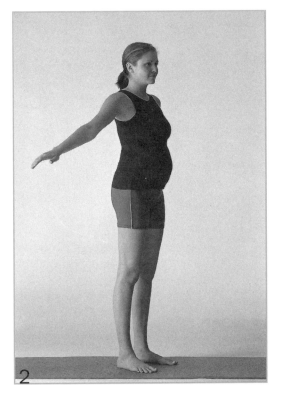

2 Keeping the shoulders down and in line with each other, continue to circle the arm round. Keep the ribcage still as you draw a circle with the arm. As the arm passes your ear, breathe out. If your ribcage moves, you are swinging too far – make the circle a little smaller.

3 Complete the circle. As your arm passes your ear breathe out and, as the arm starts to pass your leg, breathe in.

double arm circles

This movement is an advance level of the one arm circles on the facing page.

! WARNING

If one side feels a little tighter and the circle on this side is smaller, work both circles to the smaller size; this will help to bring a balance back between both sides. Start the circles small, and increase in size when you feel that both sides are working at the same level.

emphasis	mobility
visual cue	drawing a circle
repeat	5 times each way

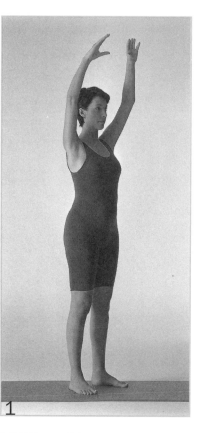

1 Stand tall with your feet apart, knees soft. Lengthen up from the top of your head to the ceiling to check that your back is correctly aligned. Breathe in and lift your left arm in front of you, then lengthen to the ceiling.

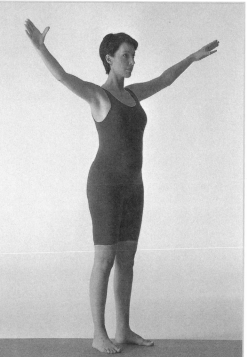

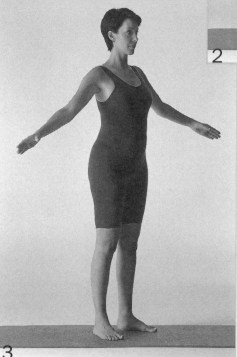

2 Keeping the shoulders down and in line with each other, continue to circle the arms round. Keep the ribcage still as you draw circles with each arm. As the arm passes your ear, breathe out. If your ribcage moves, you are swinging too far – make the circles a little smaller.

3 Complete the circles, and continue the breathing. As your arm passes your ear, breathe out; as it starts to pass your leg, breathe in.

cat/dog

The movement should be slow and continuous. Try not to overextend at the end of every end move. If you feel a tightness or pinching in the lower back, you may have tilted the pelvis up too far in the first part of the movement. Begin with small movements and gradually allow them to build in size. Do not force the movement at any time, and always keep your lower abs drawn up and in. Try to keep your neck and shoulders relaxed as you do this, with elbows slightly bent.

emphasis	mobility of the spine
visual cue	stretching like a cat
repeat	5–10 times

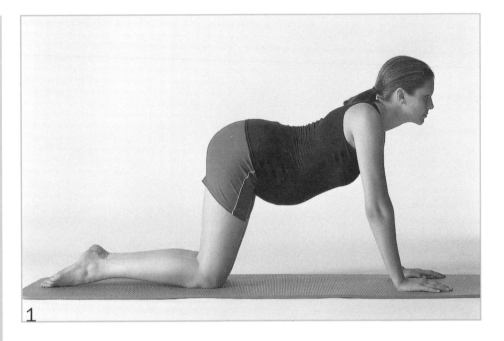

1

1 Begin on all fours; check that your hands are directly underneath your shoulders and that your knees are positioned under your hips, about hip-width apart with your feet relaxed. Draw your shoulders down and away from your ears, and lengthen your spine from the head to the tailbone, keeping your eyes down. Breathe in and gently roll your pelvis up, very gently lifting your head to look just in front of you.

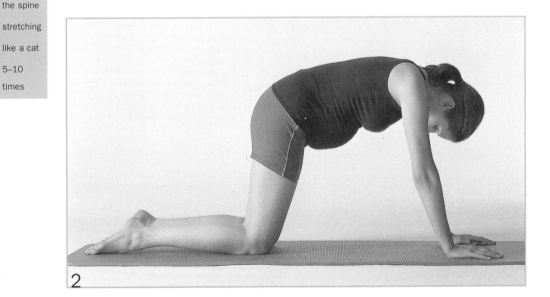

2

2 Breathe out and gently roll your pelvis down. Imagine that you have a long tail attached to your tailbone and you are dropping the tail between your legs. Let your chin slightly drop towards the chest. Gently draw your baby up towards your spine.

toy soldier

Maintain a neutral alignment as you do this – your shoulders should remain drawn down away from the ears. You may need to practise this in front of a mirror to help you check your posture. Make sure that you lengthen through the spine, especially the lower spine. Also make sure that your ribs stay just over your pelvis, your eyes are looking forwards and you can imagine you are balancing a book on your head and a thin cord is pulling you up from your head to the ceiling. Keep the movement slow and controlled.

emphasis	mobility
visual cue	air paddle
repeat	5–10 times each arm

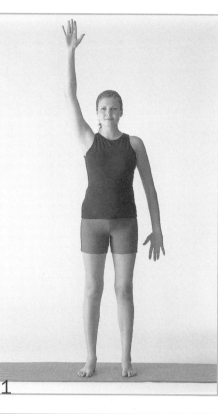

1

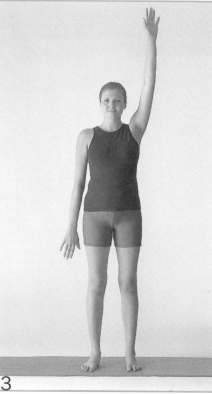

3

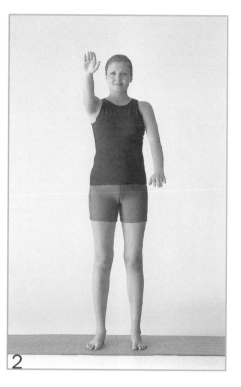

2

1 Stand tall with your feet about hip-width apart and knees soft. Breathe in, and reach your left arm to the ceiling and your right arm to the ground. Your left palm should face forwards and your right palm to the wall behind you.

2 Breathe out as you bring the lifted arm forwards and down, swapping over the positions. Try to change both arms at the same speed and without moving the torso.

3 Once the right arm has reached the ceiling and the left the ground (both should arrive at the same time), breathe in, then breathe out again as they begin to change places.

side rotation

The movement should be continuous and flowing. Let your arms relax and follow the line to the body around, trying to take the front arm a little further across the line of your body. Try not to let your head drop, and keep lengthening your spine to the ceiling. Imagine that a thin cord is pulling you up from your head towards the ceiling.

emphasis	mobility
visual cue	drawing a circle around yourself
repeat	repeat 5–10 times each side

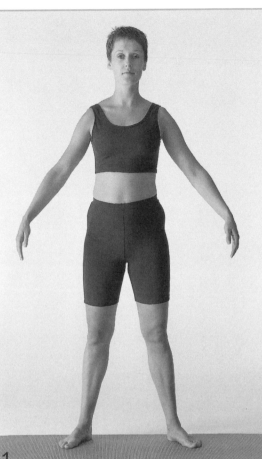

1

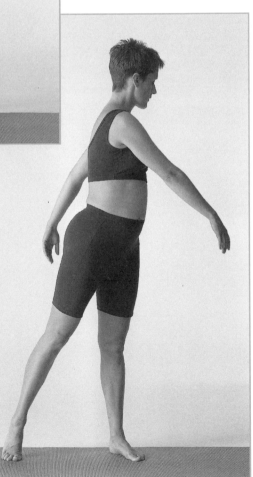

2

1 Start with your feet just wider than your hips. Draw your shoulders down and away from your ears. Allow your arms to gently float out to your side, but still keeping your shoulders down. Breathe in to prepare.

2 Breathe out and gently lift up your right heel, allowing your body to float round to the left, and letting your arms follow the line of your body.

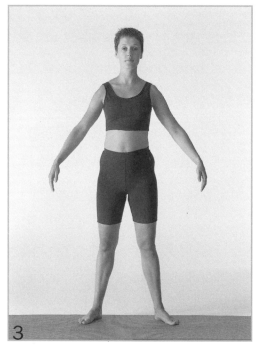

3

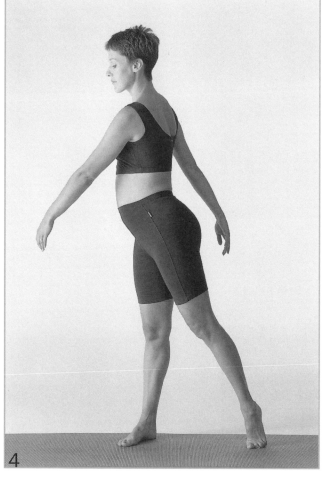

4

3 Breathe in and return to the centre, finding neutral again. Try to keep the weight evenly distributed through the feet.

4 Breathe out and gently lift your left heel, allowing your body to float round to the right again allowing your arms to follow round.

warm-up summary

The warm-up is also a time to think about neutral and bringing each exercise back to this core position. You may need to do some small exercises first to help you find neutral (see pages 32–3 on finding neutral). The warm-up is also a chance for you to think about your breathing technique (see page 34), and allowing the mind to start to work with the body.

Try to keep all the movements flowing and continuous. Repeat each exercise about five times, more if you feel that your body requires them. On some days, your body may feel tight or tired. If so, make the appropriate adjustments, in terms of number of repetitins and duration, to the warm-up exercises you choose.

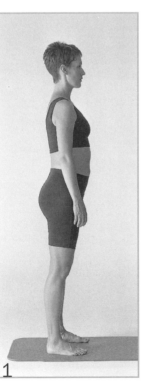

the programme

The following movements are taken from the original work by Joseph Pilates. Before you begin the programme, make sure that you are familiar with the correct levels for your stage of pregnancy and your proficiency in Pilates. See pages 38–41 to ensure that you are clear on the right level for you. Remember, you can take up Pilates at any time during pregnancy, even if you have never done it before.

push-up

Keep the movement continuous. Try to think of it as a single long, slow movement. As the size of your baby grows, this movement is going to be limited by the baby and into the third trimester may be impossible to achieve. Be careful not to strain your back and to keep the neutral alignment of all joints (see pages 32–3).

emphasis	strength
visual cue	roll into
	yourself
	and the
	baby
repeat	5 times

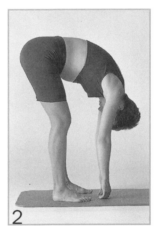

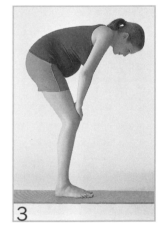

1 Stand tall in a neutral position, with feet hip-width apart and your knees relaxed. Breathe in.

2 As you breathe out, draw in the lower abdominal muscles, pulling the baby in towards the spine. Slowly start to roll the spine down, leading the roll with your head and letting the chin drop to the chest. Allow the shoulders to roll down with the body and the weight of your arms to pull you down as far as is comfortable.

3 If you cannot touch the floor without strain on your back, go to the furthest point of the roll down, bend your knees and place your hands on your thighs. Breathe out, gently draw the baby in towards your spine and gently lean forwards to place your hands on the floor.

4 Breathe out, draw the baby in towards the spine and gently lean forwards and place your hands on the floor. Walk your hands forwards on the floor as your knees bend towards the floor. Keep the movement slow, smooth and gentle. Stop walking when your knees are close to the floor and your hands are at shoulder level. Breathe in.

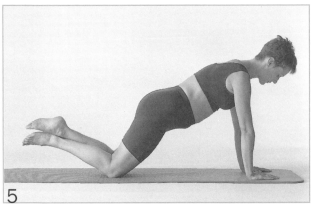

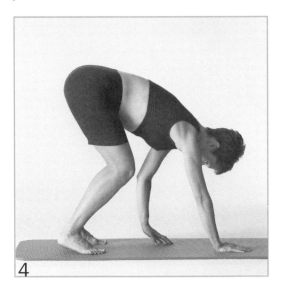

5 Breathe out and gently float your knees down onto the floor so that you are now in a box position. Cross your ankles and keep your hands and shoulders in line with each other. Imagine a line between your two hands along the floor. Breathe in, and gently lower your nose towards the line. Don't worry if you can't reach the line. Breathe out, and slowly push back up on your arms until they are fully extended, but slightly bent at the elbows.

push-up modification

If you find it difficult to execute this move, stay in this position and do three press-ups before you uncurl. This may also help if you are finding it hard to concentrate on the move as one whole move.

! WARNING

Don't straighten the arm so far that the elbow joints lock, and avoid hunching your shoulders. There should be no pressure in the lower back.

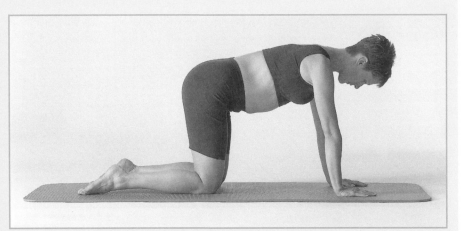

If you find the push-up part too difficult, start with a box push-up. Make sure that your hands are directly underneath your shoulders and your knees directly under your hips, maintaining a stronger base. Perform the press-up phase as before, but there is no need to cross the ankles or transer the weight forwards.

swimming

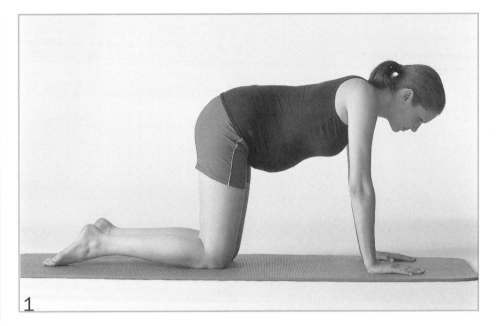

1

Keep the movement continuous and flowing, and try to maintain a neutral position of the spine, pelvis, shoulders and hips. You may not be able to lengthen the arms and legs fully without losing neutral. If so, shorten the movement, going as far as possible without coming out of neutral. Try not to lean your weight over your shoulders – keep the weight in the centre of the movement.

THE MOVEMENTS

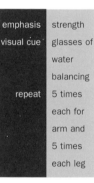

emphasis	strength
visual cue	glasses of
	water
	balancing
repeat	5 times
	each for
	arm and
	5 times
	each leg

1 Start on all fours. Check your hands are directly under your shoulders and that your knees are directly under your hips. Knees and feet should be hip-width apart and parallel. Find your neutral position on all fours, draw your shoulders away from your ears and lengthen your spine from the tip of your head to your tailbone. Allow the lower back to maintain a neutral curve, and gently roll your pelvis back and forth until you feel it is in a neutral position and that the curve in the lower back is not exaggerated, tight or uncomfortable. Lengthen your neck, and keep your eyes on the floor, being careful not to lift the head as you begin movement. Begin by finding your breathing pattern and breathe into your back and sides (see page 34). As you breathe out, draw the weight of the baby up into you, using those lower abdominal muscles to hug the baby close.

2 Breathe out as you gently extend your right arm. Don't let the arm rise above the ears and keep the shoulders level. Breathe in and slowly return your hand to the floor under your shoulder. Minimize movement through your shoulders as you lift and lower the arm.

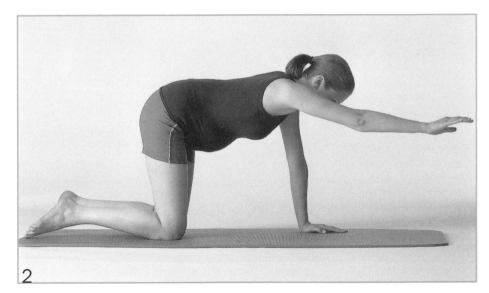

2

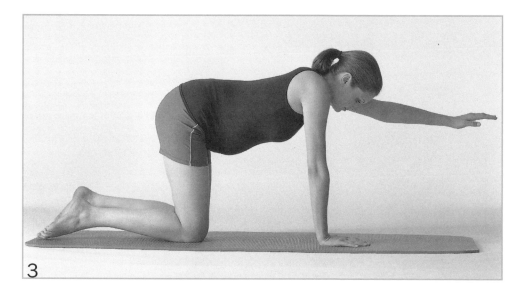

3 Breathe out and gently lengthen your left arm to the front of the room. As you breathe out, draw the baby in close. Breathe in and place the hand back on the floor. Be careful not to transfer your weight from side to side as you change arms. Continue to change arms until you have done five repetitions on each side. The challenge is to minimize the movement through the rest of the body as you change sides. Imagine that you have two very full glasses of water on each shoulder as you change sides and that you don't want to rock the glasses and spill the water.

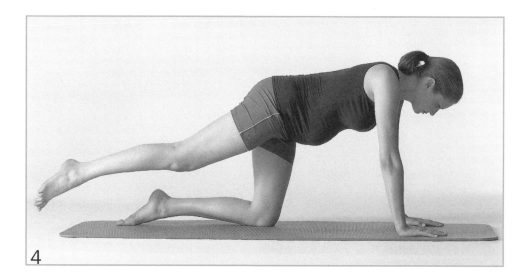

4 This time the arms stay in position and the legs move. Breathe out while lengthening the right leg out behind you. Keep the foot in contact with the floor to begin with. When you become more confident, lift the foot slightly off the floor. Breathe in and gently slide the leg back to its place beneath your hips, placing the knee back down without rocking the hips.

Breathe out and gently lengthen the left leg out behind you, breathe in and gently draw the leg back in. Remember as you breathe out to draw the baby in nice and close. Imagine you have those two very full glasses of water on your hips now. As you change sides, try to minimize the rocking movement in the hips and also to prevent one side lifting higher than the other.

roll-down/roll-up

This movement is a modification of the roll-up: concentrate on both parts of the movement being equal in speed and control. If your feet lift off the floor, you have gone too low. Feel the lengthening through the lumbar spine as you curl back and down. Try to concentrate on tucking your tailbone under when you curl down, as if you were trying to imprint your bottom into the mat.

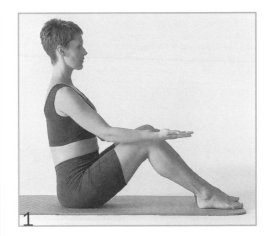

1 Start from a seated position with your arms stretched out in front of you. Sit tall as if you have a hook on the top of your head, pulling you up towards the ceiling. Slide your shoulders down and back, away from your ears. Keep your knees bent and hip-width apart and feet on the floor, in line with your knees and a comfortable distance from your body. You should be able to sit without hunching your shoulders. Imagine a hard-backed chair behind you.

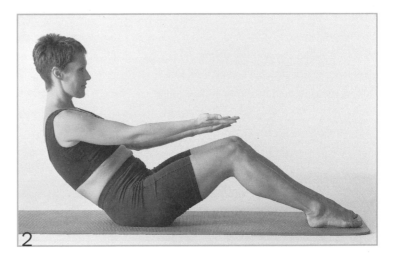

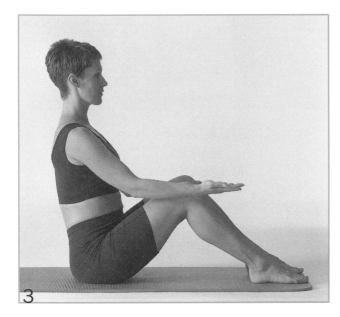

2 Breathe in, and gently lean back by tucking the pelvis under you as you roll down, while keeping your arms relaxed and floating above the knees, palms facing up. Lean back only as far as you can while keeping control of the movement. This will be determined by the flexibility of your back, the strength in your centre and the size and position of your baby. Try to make sure the lower abdominal muscles gently draw in as opposed to pushing out.

3 Breathe out, and slowly return to the upright position. Lengthening towards the ceiling again, breathe in and slowly roll back again without stopping. The roll down and up should be one long, continuous movement.

THE MOVEMENTS

roll-down/roll-up modification

As you progress
through your
pregnancy, you may
find it reassuring to
sit just forwards of
a wall or sofa to
perform this
exercise. If you feel
you are struggling to
get back up, you can
then rest against the
sofa or wall behind
you instead of going
all the way down onto
your back.

You may wish to modify this movement slightly, by placing your hands lightly under the backs of your thighs. This can provide a little assistance in helping you return to the upright position. But be careful not to pull too hard on the thighs. If you feel yourself doing this, you are going too low. This does limit how far down you can go, but is a great modification, especially as you get bigger and the weight in your centre increases. The control is more important than how far back you can go.

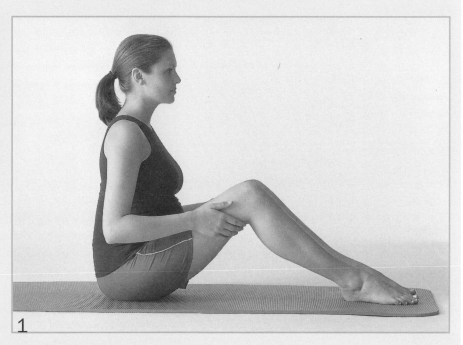

1

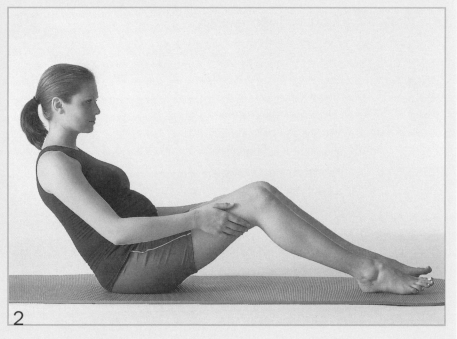

2

one-leg circles

There are two main challenges with this exercise: the first is to make sure that the space under the lower back doesn't change as you lift or lower the leg or circle the leg round; the second is to minimize the movement in the hips as you change legs, trying to keep the same amount of pressure under both hips regardless of which leg is lifted. Be careful not to rock the pelvis as you change legs or circle the leg. You may try putting your hands on top of the pelvic bones on either side of your hips to see whether you feel any movement as you change legs.

emphasis	mobility
visual cue	a 10-pence piece
repeat	5 times in each direction, each leg

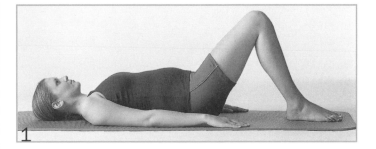

1 Lie on your back with your knees bent and feet flat. Make sure that your knees and feet are hip-width apart and that they stay parallel to each other. Place your feet comfortably close to your bottom. Find neutral of the spine and pelvis (see pages 32–3), becoming aware of the small space underneath your lower spine. It is important to focus on this, especially once you add movement. The focus will be for the space to remain the same throughout the exercise,

showing that you have maintained neutral position of the pelvis and spine. Begin by thinking about your breathing. As you breathe in, try to get your back to expand across the mat under you. As you breathe out, draw the baby in and down to the spine. Maintaining this position may be a challenge for you. Remember to time yourself and do not spend any longer than 5 minutes on your back. If you start to feel dizzy or light-headed, roll onto your side immediately.

2 If you feel ready to progress the movement, on your next out breath gently float the right leg up to a right angle. Make sure that the knee is directly above the hip with the foot in line with the knee. Place the hand on the knee and start to draw a small circle with your knee, allowing your hand to guide the knee. Imagine you are drawing a circle the size of a 10-pence piece on the ceiling. Breathe in as the knee comes in towards the centre of your body and out as it circles out and away from the body.

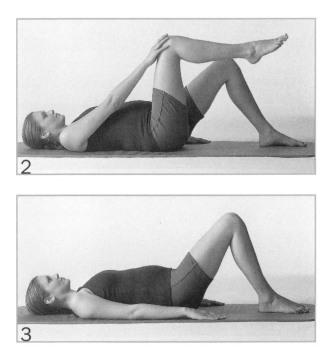

3 On your last breath out, gently float the leg back down again, placing the foot in exactly the same place it came from. Roll onto your side and rest.

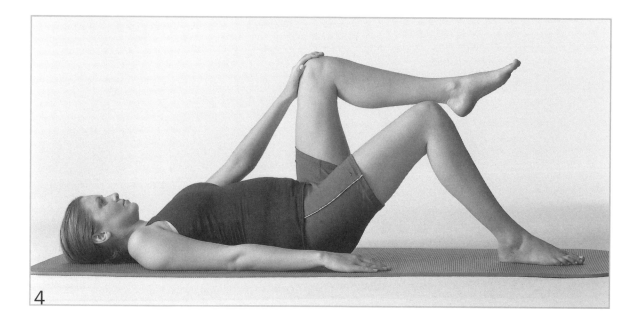

4

After a few moments, roll onto your back and find your neutral position. As you breathe out, gently float the left leg up to a right angle as before., Place your left hand on your left knee and gently start to draw a small circle with your knee. Repeat the movements as in step 2. On your last breath out, gently float the leg back down again, placing the foot in the same place it came from. Roll onto your side and rest.

one-leg circles modification

Rmember to work within a pain-free zone. If anything feels uncomfortable, first try slowing the movement down through the tight or uncomfortable part. If that does not ease the discomfort, then simply stop doing the exercise.

! **WARNING**

If you feel dizzy at any time, remember to roll over onto your side.

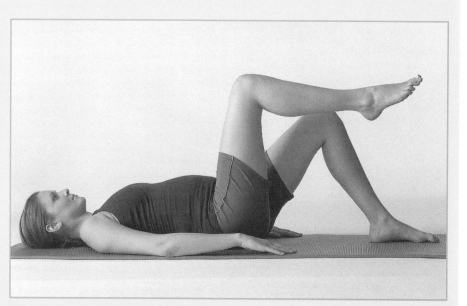

Once you become more confident with this move, try to modify it by removing the guiding hand. Remember to keep the circle small and minimize the movement in the hips. Try to feel the leg stirring all the way around inside the hip socket, and also try not to let your leg drop heavily into the hip socket.

the hundred

60

There are two main challenges with this exercise: the first is to make sure that the space under the lower back doesn't change as you lift or lower the leg; the second is to minimize the movement in the hips as you change legs. Try to keep the same amount of pressure under both hips, regardless of which leg is lifted. Be careful not to rock the pelvis as you change legs. You may try putting your hands on top of the pelvic bones on either side of your hips to see if you feel any movement under your hands as you change legs.

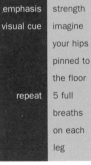

emphasis	strength
visual cue	imagine your hips pinned to the floor
repeat	5 full breaths on each leg

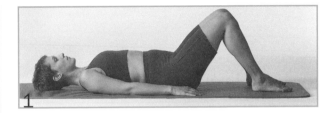

1 Lie on your back with your knees bent and feet flat. Make sure that your knees and feet are hip-width apart and that they stay parallel to each other. Place your feet comfortably close to your bottom. Find neutral of the spine and pelvis and become aware of the small space underneath your lower spine. It is important to focus on this, especially once you add movement. The focus will be for the space to remain the same throughout the exercise, showing that you have maintained neutral position of the pelvis and spine. Maintaining this position may be enough of a challenge for you. If you start to feel dizzy or light-headed, roll on to your side immediately.

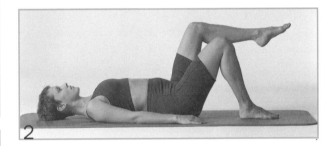

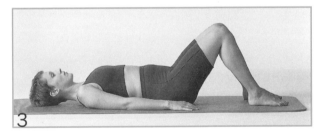

2 If you feel ready to take the movement to the next level, as you next breathe out, gently float the right leg up to a right angle, making sure that the knee is directly above the hip and the foot is in line with the knee. Continue holding the leg in this position as you continue to breathe. Try to breathe in for five counts and out for five counts until you have completed five full breaths in total.

3 On your last breath out, gently float the leg back down, placing the foot in the same place it came from. Breathe in to restabilize the pelvis and establish a neutral position.

4 As you breathe out, gently float the left leg up to a right angle as before, breathe in for five breaths and out for five breaths. On the last breath out, slowly float the leg back down, placing the foot in the same position it came from. Roll onto your side and rest.

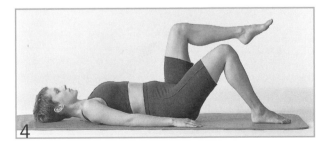

shoulder bridge

This movement is for opening and mobilizing the whole spine. Make sure that you come back to neutral each time before you imprint and start again. Pay particular attention to your knee position, and try to make sure that your knees remain parallel to each other.

emphasis	mobility and strength
visual cue	rolling paint on the floor
repeat	5 times

1 Lie on your back with your arms by your side. Think of the top of your head being pulled to one end of the room and your tailbone being stretched to the other. Find the neutral position of your pelvis and lower back (see pages 32–3). Lengthen your fingertips towards your feet to help draw your shoulders down. Breathe in to prepare for the movement.

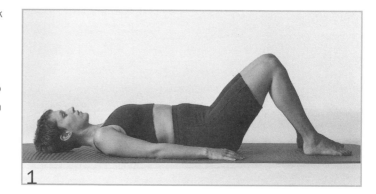

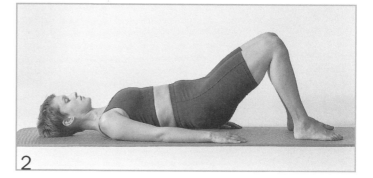

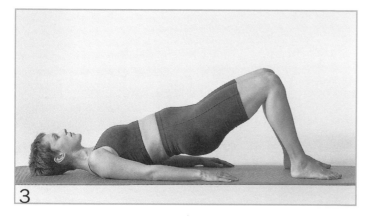

2 Breathe out, gently imprinting the lower spine into the mat. Start rolling up through the pelvis, so that the pelvis is pointing towards the ceiling. Leading with your tailbone, allow your vertebrae to lift off the floor one at time.

3 Lift your hips slowly until your body forms a slope position, resting on your shoulder blades. Try not to put pressure on the neck and shoulders. As you lift, try to focus on drawing up through the pelvic floor muscles (see page 30–1). Breathe in and gently replace the spine back down on the mat, focusing on one vertebrae at a time. Once the hips touch the floor, roll the pelvic back to neutral.

4 As you become bigger, it may be harder for you to lift your hips very far off the floor, so reduce the movement so that you just lifting the hips.

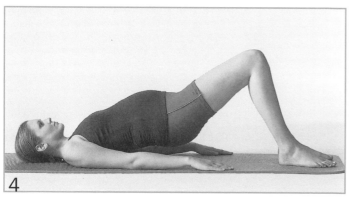

one-leg stretch

This movement challenges you to maintain neutral while extending the leg and changing legs. If you feel dizzy or light-headed at any time during the exercise, stop immediately and roll onto your side.

emphasis	strength
visual cue	toe reach
repeat	5 times on each leg

1 Lie on your back with your knees bent and feet flat. Make sure that your knees and feet are hip-width apart and that they stay parallel to each other. Place your feet comfortably close to your bottom. Find neutral of the spine and pelvis (see pages 32–3), becoming aware of the small space underneath your lower spine. It is important to focus on this, especially once you add movement. The focus will be for the space to remain the same throughout the exercise, showing that you have maintained neutral position of the pelvis and spine. Begin by thinking about your breathing. As you breathe in, try to get your back to expand across the mat under you. As you breathe out, draw the baby in and down to the spine. Maintaining this position may be a challenge. Remember to time yourself, and do not spend any longer than 5 minutes on your back. If you start to feel dizzy or light-headed, roll onto your side immediately.

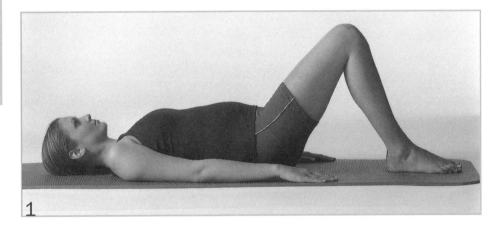

2 Place your hands on the hip bones on either side of your hips to help you focus on minimizing the movement in the pelvis as you move the legs. On your next breath out, gently slide your right leg out in front, keeping your foot in contact with the ground. Concentrate on the space under the lower back. If the size increases, do not extend the leg any further. Breathe in and slowly draw the leg back, placing the foot back where it came from.

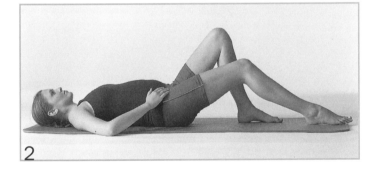

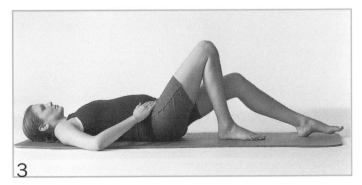

3 On your next breath out, lengthen the left leg out in front and as you breathe in slowly draw the leg back in, maintaining neutral all the time. After completing the full repetitions, roll onto your side and rest.

one-leg stretch modification

This modification requires more strength to maintain neutral. If you already find this move challenging, you may not be ready for this modification.

! WARNING

If the hollow under your lower back increases, you need to place your leg back down and continue with the first level.

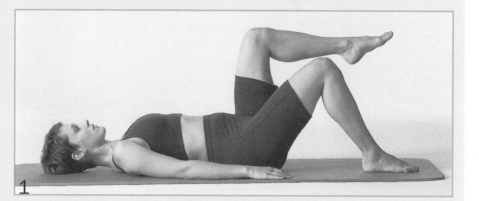

1 If you feel ready to challenge yourself a little further, the following modification takes you to the next level. Follow the directions for The Hundred movement (page 60). Lift one leg to a right angle without any shifting in the hips.

2 Once you have the right leg up at a right angle, keeping your knee directly above the hip, extend your leg to the ceiling as you breathe out. Breathe in, and return the leg to the right-angle position.

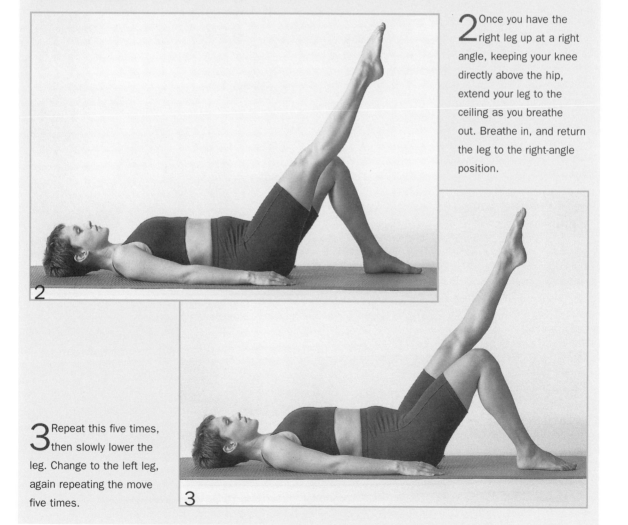

3 Repeat this five times, then slowly lower the leg. Change to the left leg, again repeating the move five times.

scissors

64

THE MOVEMENTS

There are two main challenges with this exercise. The first is to make sure that the space under the lower back doesn't change as you lift or lower the leg. The second is to minimize the movement in the hips as you change legs. Try to keep the same amount of pressure under both hips, regardless of which leg is lifted. Be careful not to rock the pelvis as you change legs. Put your hands on top of the pelvic bones on either side of your hips to see if you feel any movement under your hands as you change legs.

emphasis	strength
visual cue	dipping your toes in water
repeat	5 times for each leg

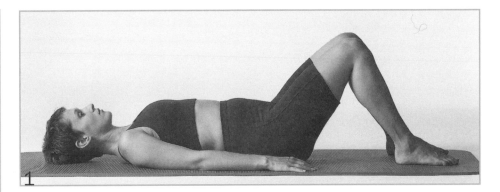

1 Lie on your back with your knees bent and feet flat. Make sure that your knees and feet are hip-width apart, parallel to each other, and that your feet are comfortably close to your bottom. Find neutral (see pages 32–3), and become aware of the small space underneath your lower spine and focus on this shape. As you add movement, this space must remain the same size; if at any time it increases, place the legs back down. Remember to roll onto your side if you feel dizzy or light-headed.

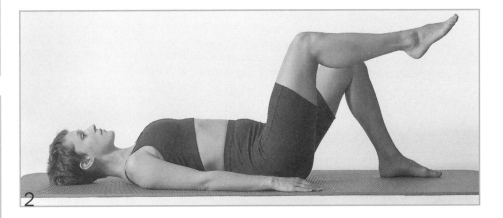

2 As you next breathe out, gently float the right leg up to a right angle, making sure that the knee is directly above the hip and the foot is in line with the knee. Breathe in.

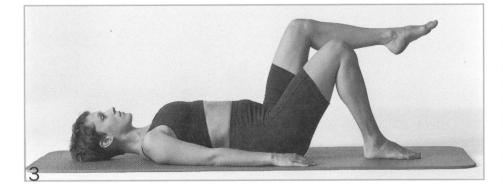

3 Breathe out, and gently the float the leg back down again, placing the foot in the same place it came from. Now breathe in to restabilize the pelvis and establish a neutral position.

4 Breathe out, and gently float the left leg up to a right angle as before. Breathe in and then out, placing the foot in the same position it came from. Continue to change the legs from right to left, focusing on minimizing the movement in the pelvis as you change legs. Roll onto your side and rest.

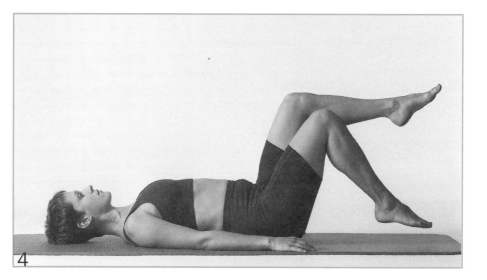

4

scissors modification

As you progress through your pregnancy, you may find it extremely difficult to lift the legs and not overarch the lower spine. The following modification allows you to continue the same movement, but takes the pressure off the lower spine.

! WARNING

If the space underneath your lower back increases or you feel any discomfort in the groin area, then rest the legs down and roll onto your side.

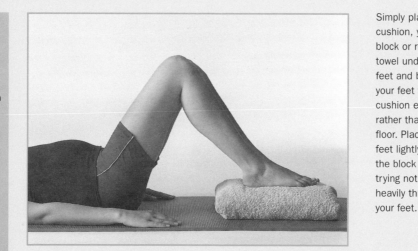

Simply place a cushion, yoga block or rolled-up towel under your feet and bring your feet to the cushion each time rather than the floor. Place your feet lightly onto the block or towel, trying not to land heavily through your feet.

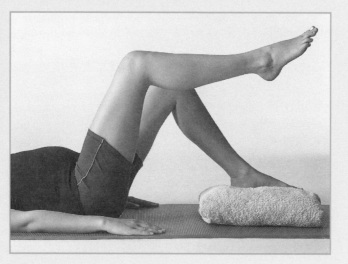

side kick

This movement challenges your balance. Progress slowly through the levels, remembering not to go too far too soon. Adjust the level and intensity with whatever stage of pregnancy you are at. This time as you breathe out, try to remember to focus on the pelvic floor muscles, drawing them up as opposed to drawing in the lower abdominal muscles. Remember as you work the pelvic floor muscles that the lower abdominal muscles will also be activated.

THE MOVEMENTS

emphasis	strength, lengthen
visual cue	long drawn arrow
repeat	5 full breaths

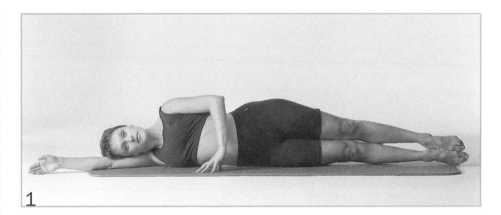

1 Lie on your right side and check that your spine is in a horizontal line. Your hips, knees, and shoulders should be in a straight line, one on top of the other. Lengthen your legs as if you were trying to touch the far wall. Place your left arm on the floor above your head, roughly in line with your baby to offer support and balance, making sure you draw the shoulders down. Maintaining this balanced position, breathe in and out. As you breathe out, try to draw up the pelvic floor (see pages 30–1).

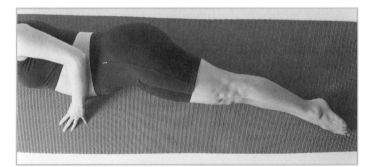

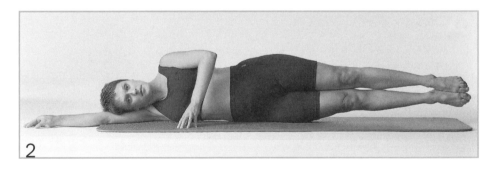

2 If you feel ready to progress and are able to balance, remaining in neutral, on your next breath out gently float both legs up about 5 inches off the floor. Maintain this lift as you breathe for five full breaths. On your last breath out, slowly lower the legs back down, maintaining control as you do so. If you feel any discomfort or pinching in your lower back at all, lower your legs to the floor immediately.

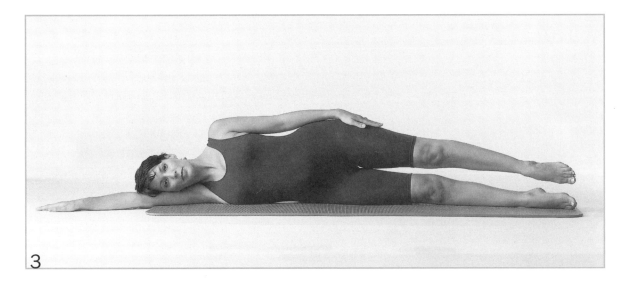

3

3 If you feel ready to progress and are able to remain neutral and balanced with the lifted legs, try this modification. Take the left hand and stretch it down along the side of your body, reaching your fingertips towards your toes. As you breathe out, gently float up the top leg only. Breathe in and lower the leg, then change to the other side.

side kick modification

Imagine that you are painting a line along the bottom of your skirting board with your big toe. Keep the hand in front for support.

! WARNING

If you feel any discomfort or pinching in the lower back or groin area, lower the legs and rest.

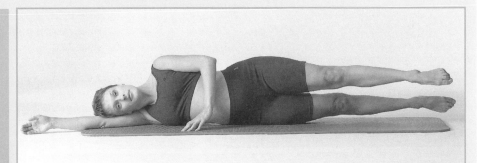

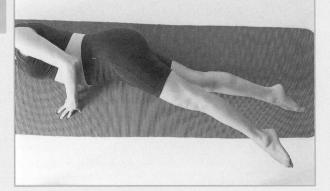

If you are able to increase the intensity, slowly lift both legs as you breathe out, breathe in and briefly hold the position. Breathe out, and slowly slide the top leg forwards. Breathe in, and gently draw it back in line with the bottom leg. Repeat three times. Lower both legs gently as you breathe out.

spine stretch

This movement is designed to help with the mobility in your spine. It should also help to ease any lower back pain, as it lengthens the muscles in the lower back. Be careful not too go too far forwards, and if you feel discomfort in the lower back, stop. Watch that your shoulders don't roll forwards and that you keep the chest as open as possible. Roll over the beach ball, but don't fold into yourself.

emphasis	strength
visual cue	roll over
	the
	beach ball
repeat	5 times

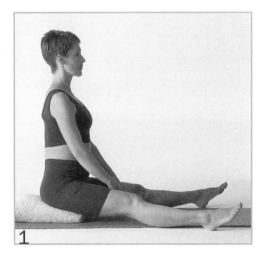

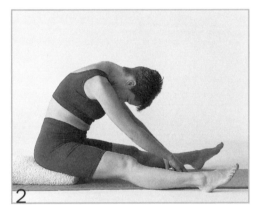

1 Sit on the edge of a folded towel, yoga block or cushion, so that you feel your weight roll forwards into your pelvis, with your legs stretched out in front of you and apart, your hands on the floor between them. Sit up tall and lengthen your spine as if a string attached to your head were drawing you up to the ceiling. Draw your shoulders down and away from your ears, allowing your chest muscles to open. Try to imagine sitting up against a hard-backed chair. Breathe in.

2 As you breathe out, draw in the lower abdominal muscles and gently start to roll forwards, as if you were rolling over a large beach ball, trying to imprint your forehead into the beach. Breathe in and slowly rewind, uncurling your spine until you are sitting upright against the imaginary hard-backed chair. Keep your hips still and in contact with the towel.

spine stretch modification 1

Keep the arms in line with your chest, keeping the shoulders down.

! WARNING

Keep the movement small to begin with.

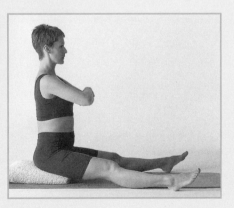

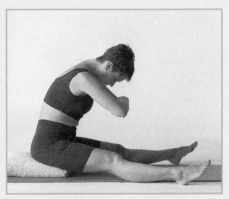

As the size of your baby grows, you may need to modify the movement. Sit tall and cross your arms so that your fingertips touch your elbows.

spine stretch modification 2

Try not to let the knees roll out as you do this exercise. If you need to, move the feet wider apart so that the knees feel more comfortable.

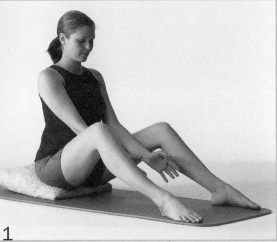

1
1 You may find it uncomfortable to sit with your legs straight, especially if your hamstrings are feeling tight. Modify the movement by bending the knees and bringing the feet close in.

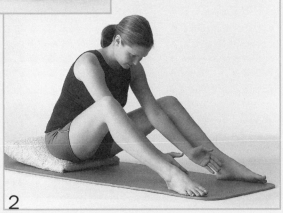

2 As you breathe out, gently curl over the beach ball (the beach ball is a lot bigger this time). Once your forearms touch the beach ball, slowly breathe in and rewind.

2

spine stretch modification 3

Remember to sit up tall at the end of each movement. Try to imagine gently rolling a ball forwards in front of you.

! WARNING

This move should be continuous, so try not to stop at the bottom of the movement.

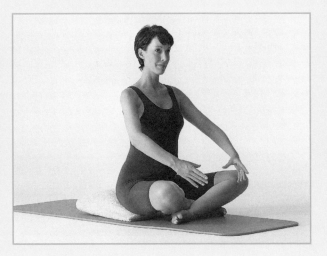

An alternative is to sit with the legs crossed. This may cause pins and needles in the legs, especially if the circulation is poor, so stretch the legs out between exercises. Try alternating which leg you cross on top.

spine twist

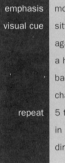

emphasis	mobility
visual cue	sitting up against a hard-backed chair
repeat	5 times in each direction

1 Sit on the edge of a folded towel, yoga block or cushion, so that you feel you weight roll forwards into your pelvis. With your legs lying stretched out in front of you and apart, cross your arms so that your fingertips are resting on your elbows. Sit up tall, and lengthen your spine as if a string attach to your head were drawing you up towards the ceiling. Draw your shoulders down and away from your ears, allowing your chest muscles to open. Try to imagine sitting up against a hard-backed chair. Breathe in.

2 Breathe out as your turn your upper body to the right side, keeping your nose and chin in line with the centre of your arms (use a watch or bracelet to help you find the centre). Keep your hips still and facing forwards as you turn.

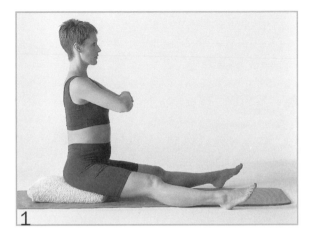

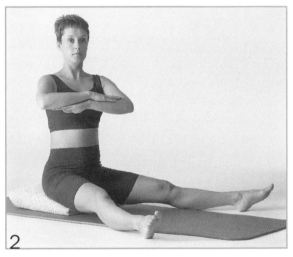

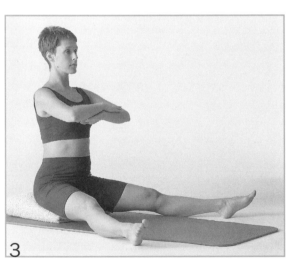

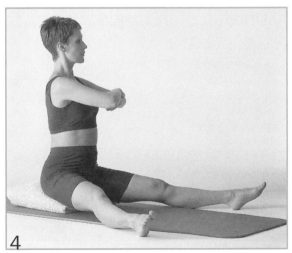

3 Breathe in and return to the centre. Lengthen your body upwards and sit tall.

4 Breathe out, and slowly turn your upper body to the left. Don't let your elbows lead you past your centre.

spine twist modification 1

Feel the muscles stretching and working in your back. As you turn and breathe out imagine you are wringing the air out of your lungs.

! WARNING

Do not sink into your back as you turn – lift out through your waist.

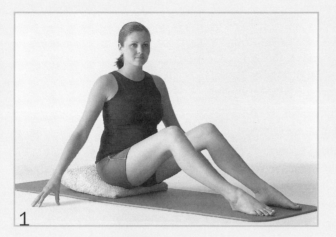

1

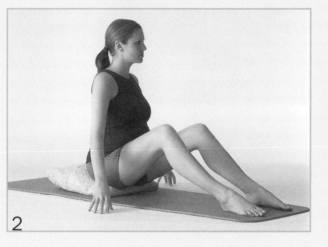

2

1 As you progress through your pregnancy and the size of the baby increases, you may find it more comfortable to modify the hand and leg positions. Bend your knees and bring your feet reasonably close to the cushion. Lengthen your arms out to the side as if you were dipping your fingers into pools of water surrounding you.

2 As you breathe out, gently turn to one side, allowing your fingers to gently flow through the water. Keep your head up and chin in line with the centre of your chest. Remember to sit tall and draw the shoulders down.

spine twist modification 2

Remember to make sure that your chin stays in line with the centre of your chest. Keep your eyes and head lifted.

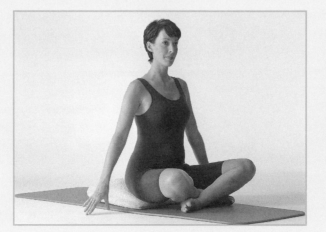

Another modification, which may become more comfortable as the baby grows, is to sit still on the cushion, but with your ankles crossed.

double arm stretch

emphasis	strength
visual cue	morning stretch
repeat	5 times

1 Lie on your back with your knees bent and feet comfortably close to you. Make sure that your feet and knees are hip-width apart and parallel to each other. Place your right hand on the centre of your ribcage, and relax your left arm down by your side. The hand over the ribcage is going to assess how much movement occurs there as you lift your other arm up and back past your head. Try to prevent the ribcage from lifting or flaring. If this happens, it means that you are losing the neutral position of the spine and that your spine is lifting slightly off the floor.

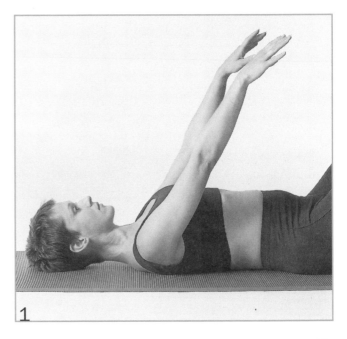

1

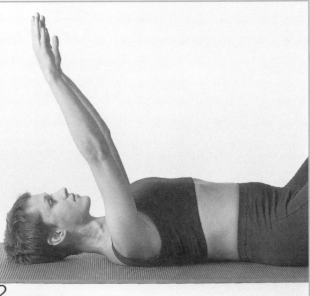

2

2 Breathe out, draw the baby in and slowly float your left arm up to a 90° angle to your body.

3 Continue breathing out, and take the arm over the head.

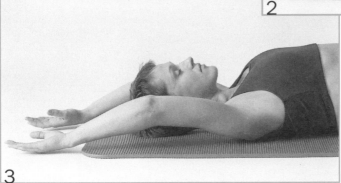

3

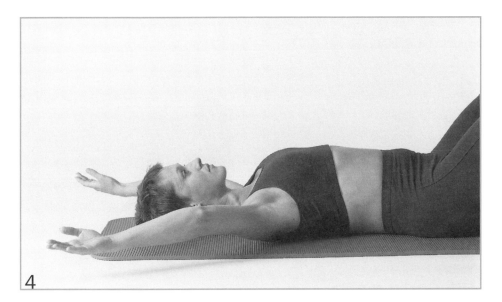

4 Breathe in and circle the arm around, hovering just above the floor.

5 Still breathing in, slowly bring the arm back to your side. Change arms, and repeat on the other side with the opposite arm now lying on your ribcage.

6 Once you have mastered the movement and are confident that you can circle the arm without coming out of neutral, you may wish to increase the challenge a little further by using both arms.

7 As the arms go over your head, be aware of the position of your pelvis and spine, and mentally check that they are still in neutral. If you find that you are unable to maintain this, simply continue with the single arm variation.

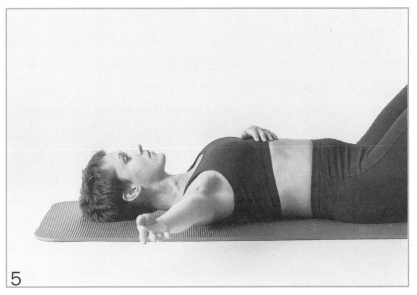

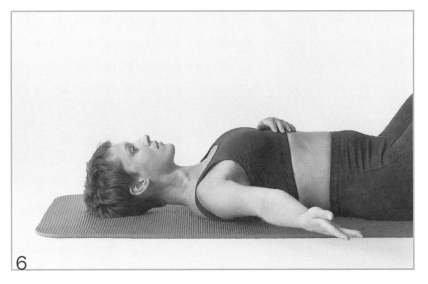

double arm stretch modification

1 As you progress through your pregnancy, you may struggle to maintain the neutral position while lifting the arms and may also find it uncomfortable to lie on your back. Sit tall on a cushion, yoga block or folded towel, lengthen the spine and keep your posture in neutral. Imagine sitting up against a hard-backed chair. Relax your arms down beside you.

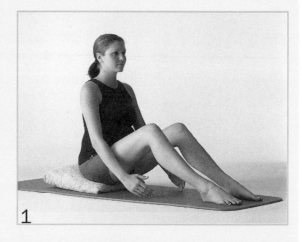

1

2 As you breathe out, slowly float your arms up to head height, concentrating on keeping the shoulders down and the chest open.

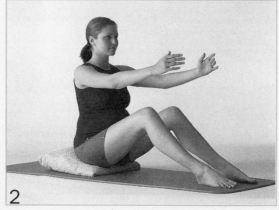

2

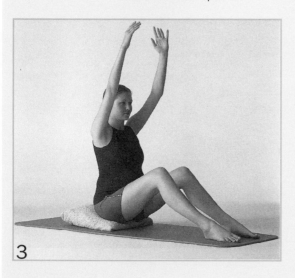

3

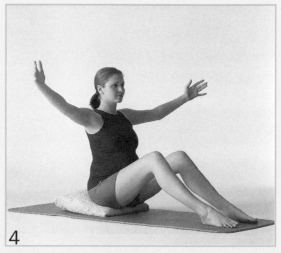

4

3 Continue breathing out, and lengthen your arms up towards the ceiling.

4 Start to breathe in, and slowly bring the arms back down to your sides. Lengthen your spine and begin again on the breath out.

leg pull prone

emphasis	strength
visual cue	coffee
	table
repeat	5 breaths
	if possible

1 Start in the box position, on all fours. Check that your hands are directly under your shoulders and that your knees are directly under your hips. Your knees and feet should be hip-width apart and parallel to each other. Lengthen your neck, and draw your shoulders away from your ears. Keep your eyes on the floor.

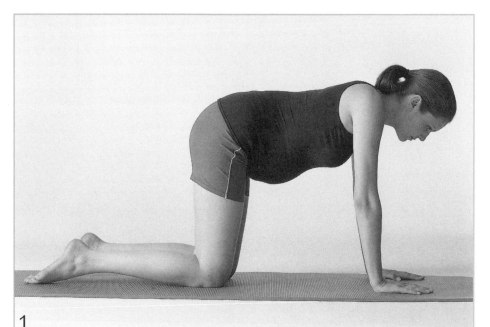

1

2 Slowly lower your elbows down to the floor. Gently roll your weight forwards, sliding the knees back, so that the fronts of your thighs starts to touch the floor. Realign the pelvis and spine, making sure that you have a neutral curve in the lower back and that the curve is not exaggerated, tight or uncomfortable. Draw your shoulders down and away from your ears and lengthen your spine. Begin by finding your breathing pattern. Breathe into your back and sides (see page 34). Breathe in, opening your back. As you breathe out, draw the baby into you using the lower abdominal muscles.

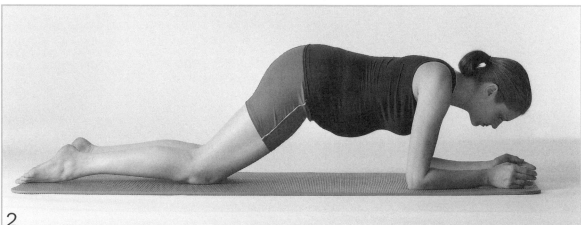

2

postnatal
movements

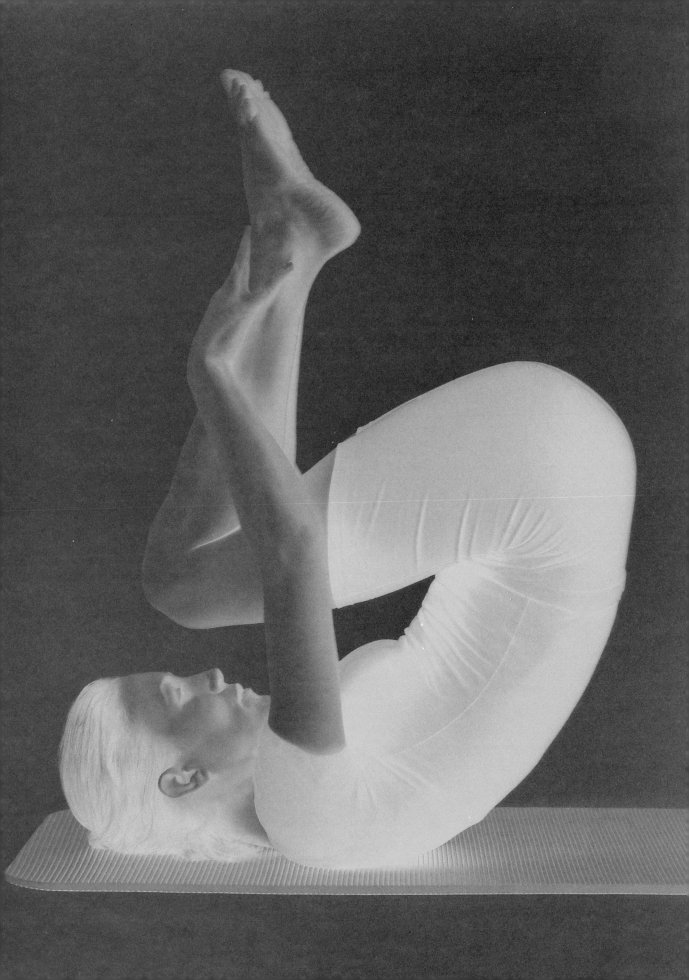

postnatal exercise

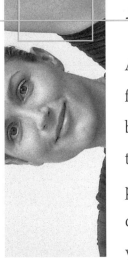

As a new mum, you may be reading this section of the book for the first time. Perhaps you have never exercised much before or have never had the chance to work with the Pilates technique. Perhaps you were unable to follow a fitness programme during your pregnancy because of health or other considerations. Whatever your situation, this book will help you to retrain your body after childbirth.

It is not advisable to return to exercise until at least six weeks after the birth and ten weeks or longer if you have had a Caesarean section or traumatic labour. You may find this a difficult time to exercise with a new baby to look after and other family and/or work commitments. But now is the best time to re-educate your body and change the way you think about your posture and the way you move.

Your body has undergone some pretty remarkable changes, not only to your posture, but to your joints and muscles as well. The following programme allows you to work through a variety of levels based on your current level of fitness. Always begin with the first level, even if you have previous experience with Pilates. This will give you time to understand how your body moves. Don't be too quick to jump to the next level.

Before you work through the following moves, take time to read the introductory chapters from pages 6–41, they will give you a better understanding of your body and the Pilates principles and technique.

We advise you to exercise regularly, but only for short sessions to begin with. For some of the exercises, we focus on the TA muscle (transverses abdominis) and sometimes on the pelvic floor muscle (see pages 30–1). If you have had a difficult childbirth and/or the pelvic floor has been damaged, you may find working the pelvis difficult at first. If this is the case, work with the TA muscle first. By engaging this muscle, you can also start to activate the pelvic floor. As the strength returns to the pelvic floor, you can start to work with this muscle independently. It is also essential that you do the pelvic floor exercises on their own without Pilates movements.

If you have already worked through this book during pregnancy, you will hopefully have an understanding of the technique and movements. The following variations and modifications are suitable for all new mothers. Work with these movements over the next few months while continuing to review moves for pregnant women. This is of benefit even to those women who have only begun working out postnatally.

Warning!

If you have had any of the following problems either before or during this pregnancy, please consult your doctor before proceeding:

- History of poor health, eg kidney or heart problems
- Raised blood pressure
- Small baby for the dates
- Abdominal pain
- Severe anaemia (low red blood cell count)
- Exhaustion
- Bleeding, spotting or excessive vaginal discharge
- Severe swelling of the hands and feet
- Feeling faint
- Diastasis Recti (separation in the linea alba) – see page 20
- Separation in the symphysis pubis – see page 22
- Prolapse

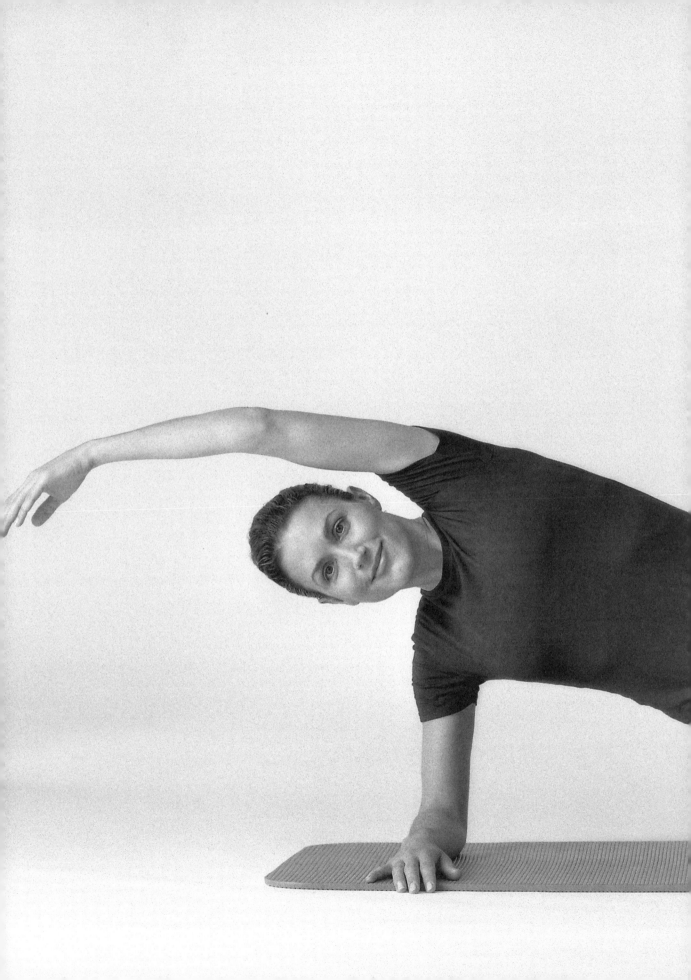

finding the right level

Improving your posture and strengthening the core muscles necessary for you to achieve your pre-pregnancy level of health and fitness are possible for every new mother, regardless of whether you already a devotee of Pilates or not. All you need to do is find the right level. The following exercises will promote a quick recovery, especially of the pelvic floor, but they will also improve general muscle tone and overall abdominal strength.

Which level for you?

Follow level one if you can answer yes to the following questions:

1. Do you still have any bleeding, spotting or excessive vaginal discharge?
2. Do you still have more than two fingers' separation in the linea alba (pages 22–3)?
3. Do you still have slight separation in the symphysis pubis (see page 22)?
4. Are you a newcomer to Pilates?
5. Do you have a medical condition which may be affected by exercise?

Follow level two if you can answer yes to the following questions:

1. Have you been doing Pilates exercises during your pregnancy?
2. Have your abdominals realigned and there is less than two fingers' gap (see pages 22–3)?
3. Do you have no abnormal bleeding or discharge?
4. Are you able to work the pelvic floor muscles?

Follow level three if you can answer yes to the following questions:

1. Have you been doing Pilates postnatally for more than two months?
2. Do you have an understanding of levels one and two?
3. Can you maintain neutral without any problems?
4. Do you have a good understanding of the Pilates technique of breathing and connecting with your centre.?

Do this for 2–3 months , then come back to this section and reassess your level.

Movement	Emphasis	Level one	Level two	Level three
Push up	Strength	1, 2, 3	1–9	1–9
Swimming	Strength	1, 2, 3	1, 2, 3	Modification
Roll-up	Strength and mobility	1, 2	1, 2	Modification
The hundred	Strength	1	1, 2, 3, 4	1, 2, 3, 4
One leg stretch	Strength	1	2	2
Spine stretch	Mobility	1, 2	1, 2	1, 2
Leg pull prone	Strength	1	1	2
Shoulder bridge	Mobility and strength	1, 2, 3	1, 2, 3	1-4
Side kick	Strength	1	1, 2	1, 2, 3, 4
Rolling back	Mobility	1, 2, 3	1, 2, 3	Modification
Spine twist	Mobility	1, 2	1, 2	Modification
Side bend	Strength	1, 2	1, 2, 3	Modifications 1–3

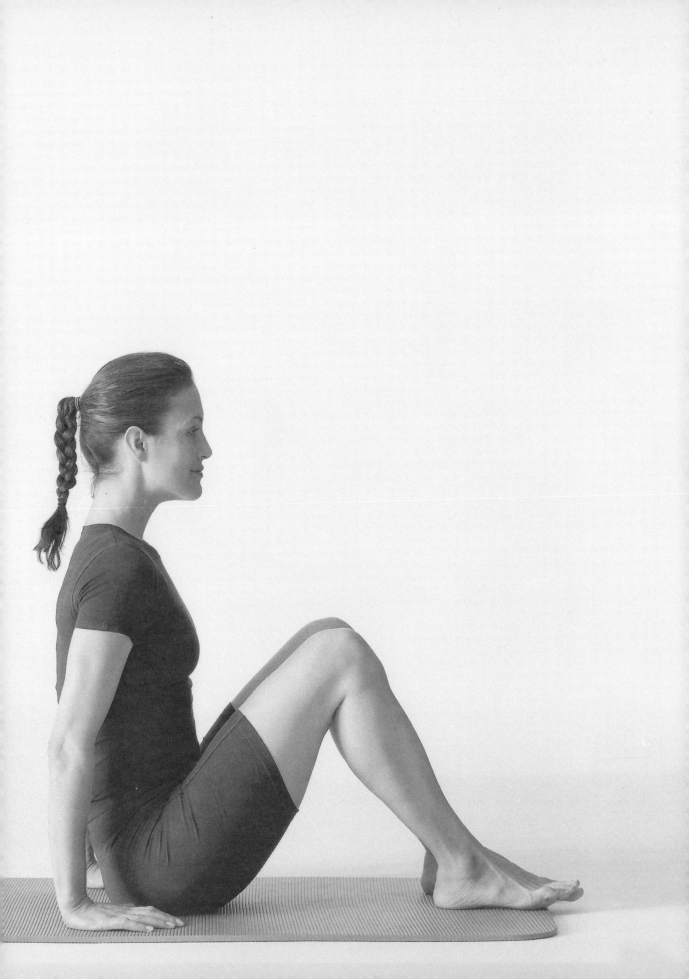

push-up

Keep the movement continuous. Try to think of it as a single long, slow movement. Be careful not to strain your back, and try to keep the neutral alignment of all the joints (see pages 32–3).

emphasis	strength
visual cue	roll into yourself
repeat	5 times

1 Stand tall in a neutral position, with feet hip-width apart, knees relaxed. Breathe in.

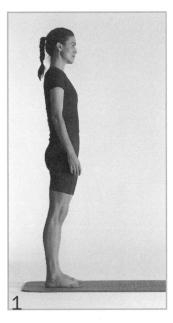

2 As you breathe out, draw in the lower abdominal towards the spine. Slowly start to bend over, rolling the spine down as you do so. Lead this movement with your head, then let the chin drop to the chest. Allow the shoulders to roll over and the weight of your arms to carry you down as far as you can without losing control. Relax and gently bend the knees as you curl down to the floor. Pay attention to your hips and, if you feel that they are pushing out behind you, bend your knees a bit more and don't go so low. It should feel as though you are folding into yourself.

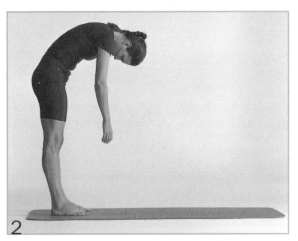

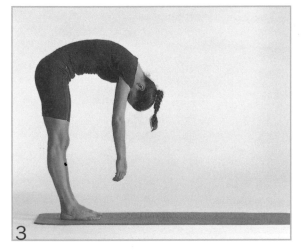

3 As you roll down, try to go as far as you can without forcing the stretch. If you feel any uncomfortable strain on your back, bend your knees slightly to release the stress. As you reach the end of the movement, breathe in and prepare to move into the press-up. If you cannot touch the floor, go to the furthest point of the roll down, bend your knees and place your hands on your thighs. Breathe out, drawing up the lower abdominals.

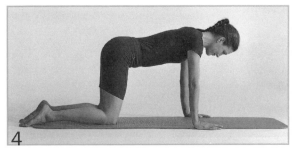

4 Gently lean forwards, and place your hands on the floor, walking your hands forwards. Keep the movement slow, smooth and gentle, as if you are trying to be as silent as possible. Stop walking the hands when your knees are under your hips and you are in a box position. Breathe in.

5 Keep your hands and shoulders in line with each other. Imagine a line between your two hands. Breathe in, and gently lower your nose towards the line. Don't worry if you can't go all the way down.

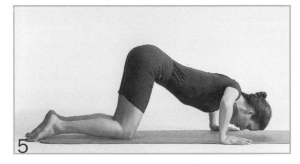

6 Breathe out and slowly push back up on your arms until they are fully extended, with your elbows slightly bent.

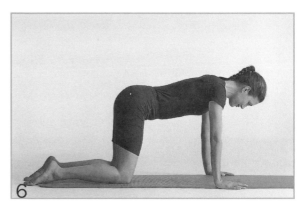

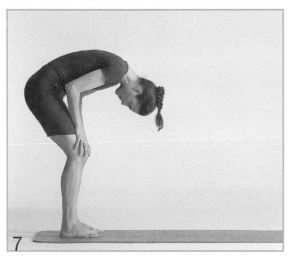

7 Breathe out, and slowly rewind the whole movement, coming back into the roll position with your hands on your thighs, knees bent and feet hip-width apart.

8 Continue to rewind, allowing the pelvis to return to a neutral position. Think of the spine as a lift going up through the levels one by one, stacking the vertebrae one at a time.

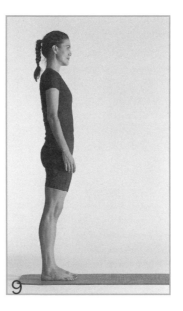

9 Finally come up to a standing neutral position, making sure that your weight is evenly planted through the feet and that your shoulders are down and relaxed. Breathe in, and prepare to start the movement once more.

swimming

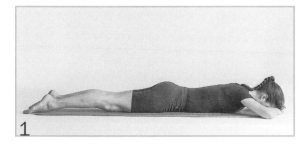

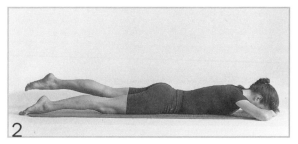

The speed of the movement should be slow and controlled. Try to lift both legs to the same height. If when lifting the leg, you struggle to keep the space under the belly button and/or the hips still, stay with the first level, concentrating on holding neutral, breathing and drawing up the centre. If you are breastfeeding or feel any stress or pain in the lower back, you may find it difficult or uncomfortable to lie flat. In these cases, read pages 50–4 to try a variation on all fours.

1 Lying face down, form a diamond shape with your arms by bending your elbows and resting your forehead on your hands. Lengthen your body through the neck and spine, and draw the shoulders down and away from your ears. Stretch your legs behind you, keeping them hip-width apart. Begin with your breathing. As you breathe out, draw up the lower abdominal muscles, creating a very small space between your belly button and the floor. Be careful not to clench your bottom or lift your hips off the floor as you do this.

2 Breathe out and lift and lengthen your right leg out behind you. Try to focus on minimizing the movement in the pelvis. Imagine a spirit level across your bottom and, as you lift the leg, don't let the bubble in the middle of the level move. Try to keep the small space between your belly button and the floor.

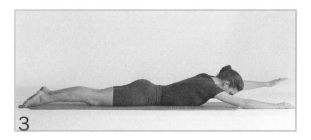

3 Breathe in and slowly lower the leg, again without moving the 'spirit level'. Breathe out and lift the left leg.

emphasis	strength
visual cue	reaching with the toes
repeat	5 times each leg

advanced swimming

Try to keep the movement smooth and continuous. You should only be lifting a few inches off the floor. Keep your eyes looking down.

! WARNING

Try not to clench the bottom. Stop and rest if you feel any discomfort or tightness in the lower back.

If you wish to challenge yourself further, try lifting the opposite arm as you lift the leg. Make sure you lift the arm and the leg to the same height, keeping the shoulders down and relaxed.

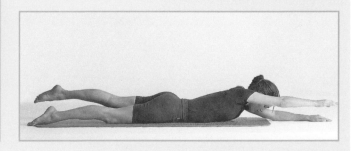

roll-up

This movement is a modification of the roll-up. In this modified version, concentrate on both parts of the movement being equal in speed and control. If your feet lift off the floor, you have gone too far back, too low. Feel the lengthening through the lumbar spine as you roll back. Try to concentrate on tucking your tailbone under you as you curl back, as if were imprinting your bottom into the mat.

emphasis	strength
visual cue	creating a C-shape in the lower back
repeat	5–10 times

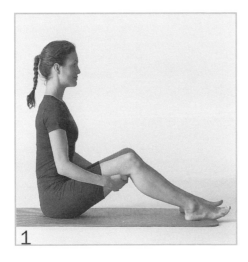

1 Start from a seated position with your knees bent and feet hip-width apart. Place your hands behind your thighs to give you assistance. Try not to pull too hard on the thighs. Sit tall as if you have a string attached to the top of your head, pulling you up towards the ceiling. Slide your shoulders down and back, away from your ears. Keep your knees bent and hip-width apart. Make sure that your feet remain in line with your knees and a comfortable distance from your body. You should be able to sit without hunching your shoulders. Imagine a hard-backed chair behind you.

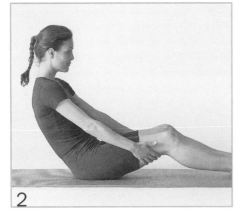

2 Breathe in and roll back by tilting the pelvis under. Roll down to a point where you feel you can keep control of the movement. This will be determined by the flexibility of your back and the strength in your centre. Breathe out and slowly return to the seated position. Stretch tall as you sit up and return to the top of the move.

roll-up modification

Remember, the control is more important than how far you can roll back. Concentrate on both parts of the move being equal in speed, effort and control. If your feet lift off the floor, you have gone too low. If you feel any tightness or discomfort in the lower back, stop and rest.

Try to remove the hands from the thighs as you do this move. This will increase the distance you can travel and also challenge you more on the return to the seated position.

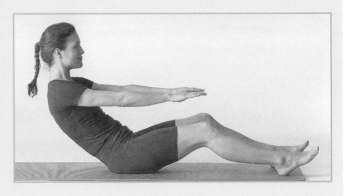

the hundred

Try to make sure that the space under the lower back does not change in size. Also try to minimize the rocking and movement in the hips as you lift your legs, keeping the weight even throught both your hips.

emphasis	strength
visual cue	imagine your hips pinned to the floor
repeat	5 full breaths on each leg

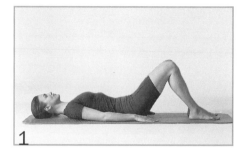

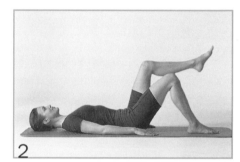

1 Lie on your back with your knees and feet hip-width apart and parallel to each other. Find neutral of the spine and pelvis (see pages 32–3). Focus on the space under your lower back, trying to keep the space the same size while you execute the movement. Just maintaining neutral and breathing may be enough of a challenge for you.

2 If you feel ready to try the next level, as you next breathe out, float the right leg up to a right angle so the knee is directly above the hip. Hold the leg in this position for five full breaths.

3 On your last breath out, gently float the leg back down, placing the foot back in the same position it came from. Check that you are still in neutral.

4 On your next out breath, repeat the above three stages, lifting the left leg, and hold for five breaths.

one-leg stretch

This movement challenges you to maintain neutral while you are extending the leg and changing legs.

emphasis	strength
visual cue	toe reach
repeat	5 times with each leg

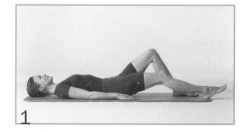

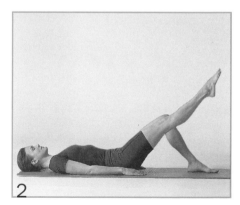

1 Lie on your back with your knees bent and feet flat. Find neutral. As you breathe out, gently slide your right leg out in front of you, only extending as far as you can without losing neutral. Breathe in, and slowly draw the leg back in. Repeat with the other leg.

2 Place your hands on the bones on either side of your hips to help you focus on minimizing movement in the pelvis. On the next breath out, gently slide your right leg out in front, keeping your foot in contact with the floor. Concentrate on the space under the lower back. If it increases, do not extend the leg any further. Breathe in, and slowly draw the leg back, placing the foot back where it came from. Repeat with the other leg.

spine stretch

This movement increases spine mobility. It should also help to ease lower back pain as it lengthens out the muscles in the lower back. Be careful not too go too low and stop if you feel discomfort in the lower back. Watch that your shoulders don't roll forward and that you keep the chest as open as possible. Roll over the beach ball but don't fold into yourself.

emphasis	mobility
visual cue	rolling over a beach ball
repeat	5–10 times

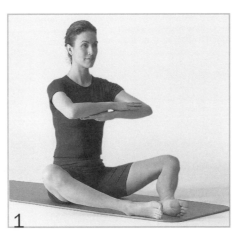

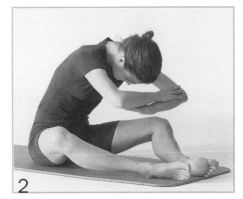

1 Sit upright with your legs in front of you, feet together and arms crossed so that your fingers touch your elbows. Sit up tall, lengthening your spine as if a string were drawing you up towards the ceiling. Draw your shoulders down and away from your ears, allowing your chest muscles to open. Try to imagine sitting up against a hard-backed chair. Breathe in.

2 As you breathe out, draw in the lower abdominal muscles and gently start to roll forwards, as if you were rolling over a large beach ball. As your forehead imprints into the beach, breathe in and slowly rewind your previous movements until you reposition your spine against the imaginary hard-backed chair. Keep your hips still and in contact with the floor.

leg pull prone (plank)

Try not to create tension in the neck and shoulders. Keep your breathing slow and relaxed. Focus on maintaining neutral.

emphasis	strength
visual cue	table top
repeat	5–10 breaths

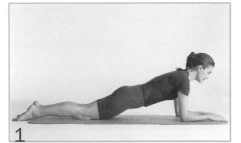

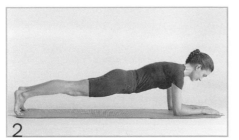

1 Resting on your forearms shoulder-width apart, gently roll your weight forwards while sliding your knees back, so that the fronts of your thighs start to touch the floor. Find neutral, making sure that you have a small curve in the lower back. Relax your shoulders and breathe. As you breathe out, try to draw in your centre.

2 If you wish to increase the intensity, gently press your toes into the floor and lengthen your heels away. As you do this, gently float up your knees. Your hips should be the same height as your shoulders. Try to hold this position for five full breaths.

shoulder bridge

This movement is for opening and mobilizing the whole spine. Make sure that you come back to neutral each time, before you imprint and start again. Pay attention to your knee position, and try to make sure that your knees remain parallel to each other at all times.

emphasis	mobility and strength
visual cue	rolling paint on the floor
repeat	5 times

1 Lie on your back in neutral with your arms by your side. Think of the top of your head pulling you to the other side of the room and your tailbone stretching you to the oppsite wall. Draw the shoulders down and breathe in to prepare for movement.

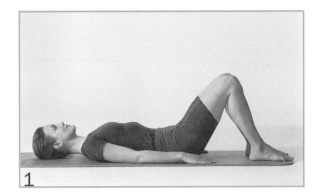

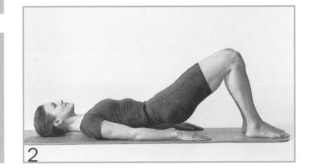

2 Breathe out, gently imprinting the lower spine into the mat. Start rolling up through the pelvis, so that it is pointing towards the ceiling. Leading with your tailbone, allow your vertebrae to lift off the floor one at time.

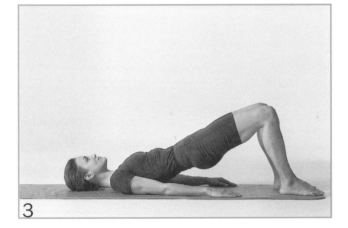

3 Lift your hips up, taking them to the height where your body forms a slope and you are resting on your shoulder blades. Try to make sure that your shoulders stay relaxed. This time, instead of focusing on your lower abdominal muscles, as you breathe out draw up on the pelvic floor (see pages 30–1). As you breathe in, gently begin to place the vertebrae back down on the mat, trying to focus on one vertebrae at a time as you trickle the spine back down. Once your hips touch the floor, gently roll the pelvis back to neutral.

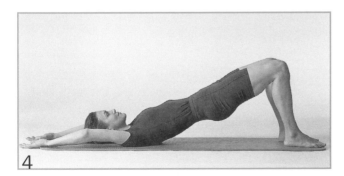

4 If you feel you are ready for a little more of a challenge, at the top of the movement stretch your arms behind you and breathe in. As you breathe out, roll back down, bringing the arms slowly over with you. As your hands touch the floor beside you, your hips should touch the floor at the same time.

side kick

This movement challenges your balance, so progress slowly through the levels, remembering not to go too far too soon. Reduce the level and intensity when you feel that you are losing that control. This time as you breathe out, try to remember to focus on the pelvic floor muscles and drawing them up, as opposed to the lower abdominal muscles and drawing them in. Remember as you work the pelvic floor muscles that the lower abdominal muscles will also be activated.

emphasis	strength
visual cue	lengthen, long drawn arrow
repeat	5 full breaths

1 Lie on your right side and check that your spine, hips, knees and shoulders are in a horizontal line. Lengthen your legs as if you were trying to touch the far wall. Place your left arm on the floor above your head, roughly in line with your belly button, to offer support and balance. Draw the shoulders down. Maintain the balance position and breathe. Focus on the pelvic floor as you breathe out.

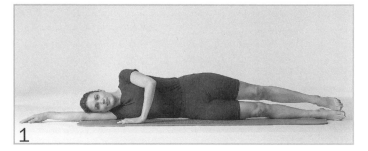

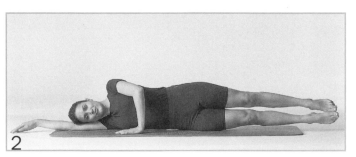

2 If you feel ready to progress and are able to balance while remaining in neutral, on your next breath out, gently float both legs up about 5 inches off the floor. Maintain this lift as you breathe for five full breaths. On your last breath out, slowly lower the legs back down, maintaining control as you do so.

4 If you feel ready to progress and are able to balance with the legs lifted, try this modification. Take the left arm and stretch it down the side of your body, reaching your fingertips towards your toes. Continue to breathe in this balanced position.

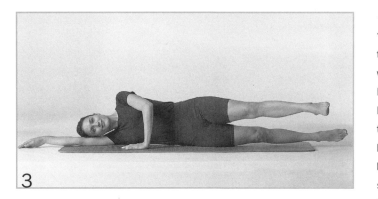

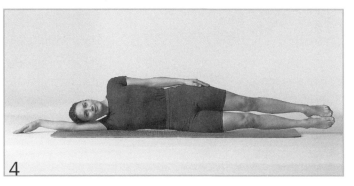

3 Once you are able to balance, try this next level, which adds in a kick. Keeping the bottom leg on the floor, lift the top leg up to hip height. As you breathe out, gently slide the leg forwards, as if you were painting a line along the skirting board with your toes. As you breathe in, bring the leg back, but don't allow it to relax on top of the bottom leg.

rolling back

Be patient and gentle with your spine until you feel that rolling becomes natural and you can return to the seated position with ease. If you have any back problems, this exercise may not be suitable. Stop if you feel any discomfort.

emphasis	mobility
visual cue	rocking chair
repeat	5–10 times

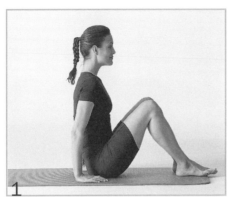

1 Sit tall, imagining a string pulling the crown of your head to the ceiling. Bend your legs with both feet together on the floor and your hands beside you.

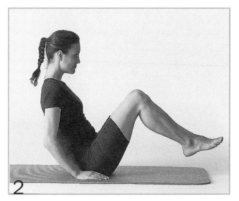

2 Taking a slow breath in, curl your pelvis forwards and start to roll back, keeping your chin close to your chest and your spine curled.

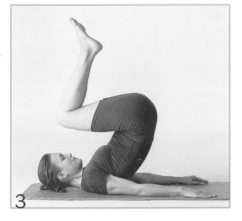

3 Gently roll back only as far as your shoulders. As you begin to roll up, use your arms to assist you in returning to an upright position by gently pressing them into the floor. Keep the abdominals drawn in and begin to breathe out slowly. Try to create the same movement as a rocking chair. Complete the breath as you return to the seated position, and lengthen your spine to the ceiling. Aim to make the roll as smooth as possible.

rolling back/down modification

Try not to land down hard on the feet or use the legs to move you. The movement should be smooth and continuous.

! WARNING

Do not roll back onto your head or neck – just to the shoulder blades.

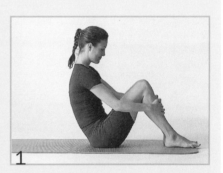

1 Once you have mastered the art of rolling, try to take away the help of the arms. Place your hands on your shins.

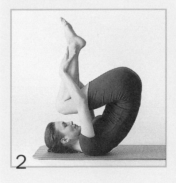

2 As you roll, keep the hands on the shins, and try to keep the space between your chest and thighs the same and the space between your bottom and feet the same.

spine twist

This movement works on the mobility of upper back. Be careful not to turn too far, and concentrate on sitting tall. As you breathe out, draw in the lower abdominals. Throughout this book we have given you many variations for this move, including those for the upper body position and the lower body position. Try to mix and match these until you find a position in which you are able to sit tall and maintain control.

emphasis	mobility
visual cue	rotation
repeat	5–10 times

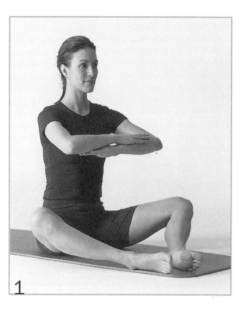

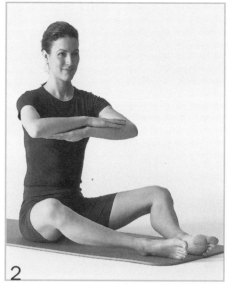

1 Sitting tall with your legs in front of you and feet together, cross your arms so that your fingertips are resting on your elbows. Sit up tall, and lengthen your spine as if a string on your head were pulling you up towards the ceiling. Draw your shoulders down and away from your ears, allowing your chest muscles to open. Breathe in.

2 Breathe out as your turn your upper body to the right. Keep your nose and chin in line with the centre of your arms (use a watch or bracelet to help you find centre). Keep your hips still and facing forwards as you turn. Breathe in, and return to the centre, lengthening your body and sitting tall. Breathe out, and slowly turn to the left side.

spine twist modification

You may wish to sit on a yoga block or towel as shown earlier in the book, especially if you are finding it difficult to sit tall. Try to keep the movement smooth and continuous. If you find holding the arms up difficult, revert to the modifications shown for this move earlier in the book (pages 70–1 and 74).

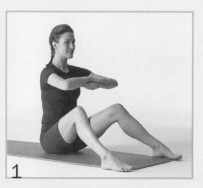

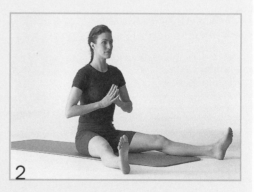

1 Another modification to the spine twist is to bend the knees and place the feet on floor.

2 If you find it difficult to maintain the centre while rotating, try to bring your hands together in a praying position. Place your thumbs onto your sternum (chest bone).

side bend

Make sure that the hips remain aligned one on top of the other throughout the exercise, being careful not to roll forwards or back. Gently place the hips down, barely touching the floor. Keep the strength of the move in your centre and not in the shoulder.

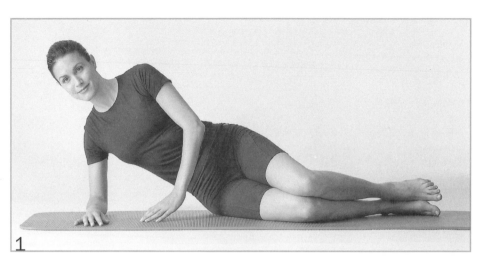

1

emphasis	strength
visual cue	stretching
	over a big
	ball
repeat	5–10

1 Start in a side line reclining position on the floor with the knees bent and the hips stacked one on top of the other. Place the right forearm on the mat, and draw your weight out of your right shoulder. Place the left hand on the floor in front of you.

2 As you breathe out, lift your hips off the floor. Only lift them to a height where you can keep your control and balance. Breathe in as you slowly lower yourself back to the start position.

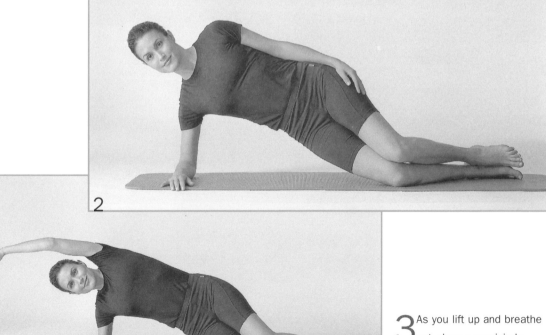

2

3

3 As you lift up and breathe out, draw a semicircle through the air, continuing to stretch the arm until you feel that your body is fully extended.

side bend modification

This movement builds strength in the torso. Challenge yourself by the height to which you lift. Make sure you don't lose the neutral line by lifting the hips too high.

1 Lie on your right hip with your right hand and elbow on the mat beneath you. Make sure that the hips are aligned and draw the weight out of the right shoulder. Bend your left leg and place it in front of your right leg, which should be straight. Relax the shoulders and open the chest.

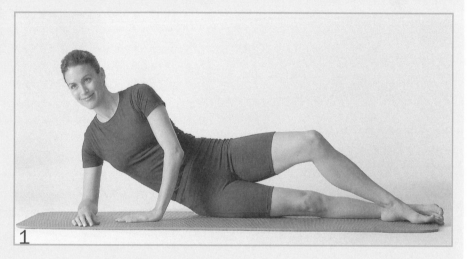

1

2 Breathe out as you lift the right hip off the floor. Gently press the left foot into the floor to help stabilize you. Breathe in and slowly lower the hips back down, barely touching the floor.

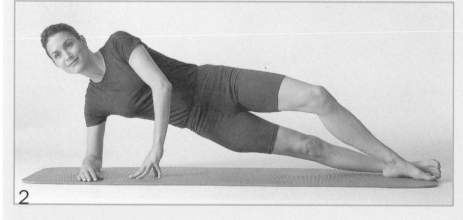

2

3 As you lift up and breathe out, the left arm draws a semi-circle through the air. Continue to stretch the arm until you feel that your body is fully extended.

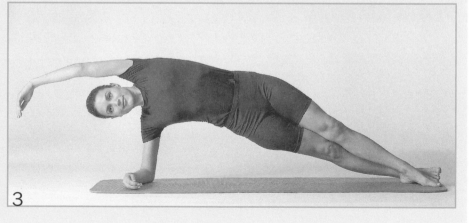

3

useful organizations

The Pilates Institute
Wimborne House, 151–155 New North Road, London, N1 6TA
Telephone: 020 7253 3177
www.pilates-institute.co.uk

Association of Breastfeeding Mothers
PO Box 207, Bridgwater, Somerset, TA6 7YT
Telephone: 020 7813 1481

Association for Postnatal Illness
25 Jerdan Place, London, SW6 1BE
Telephone: 020 7386 0868

Maternity Alliance
45 Beech Street, London, EC2P 2LX
Telephone: 020 7588 8582

Meet-a-Mum Association (MAMA)
14 Willis Road, Croydon, Surrey, CRO 2XX
Telephone: 020 8771 5595

National Childbirth Trust (NCT)
Alexandra House, Oldham Terrace, London, W3 6NH
Telephone: 020 8992 8637

Parentline
Endway House, The Endway, Hadleigh, Benfleet, Essex, SSN 2AN
Helpline: 01702 559900
Office: 01702 554782

index

acknowledgments

I would like to thank all my team at the Pilates Institute UK, Malcolm Muirhead, Yolande Green and Nuala Coombs, and all the others without whose incredible dedication and help we would not be able to promote Pilates in all its formats and reach all the parts of the world we do. Of all the people who have influenced my teaching and understanding of what Pilates can do for all of us, I would really like to thank Judith Aston who brought her fabulous technique, Aston Patterning, to the UK, trusting us with passing on her knowledge and whose technique is now a big part of Pilates. With our friends in the medical world being part of the daily dialogue, a Pilates Instructor can now be better equipped to deal with the needs of our clients. This book is dedicated to all the future mothers who I hope will use this information to train for the birth of their child, and the months, and years, afterwards.

Michael King

As Michael always used to say about the first book he wrote, it's like having a baby, nine months of stress and worry, followed by a painful period, but quickly forgotten and replaced with joy when you hold the end product in your hand, full of pride at what you have achieved. Well I think no truer words could be said about writing this book. As with any project it would not be possible without the support of family, friends and colleagues. I know that we would both like to thank Malcolm, Nuala and the whole team at the Pilates Institute for their suppport, and I would personally like to thank my mum, dad, my brother Denzil and sister Bev for their continuous support throughout my career, without whom I could not have reached my goals. I would also like to thank my close friends, Pete, Hannah, Michele and Claire for putting up with me being sometimes unbearable whilst writing this book, and finally to my friends at Bramston who also gave me support and encouragement.

Yolande Green